| | |
|---|---|
| Introduction | 5 |
| About Me | 13 |
| Changing Your Mind! | 15 |
| Prevention and Treatment | 42 |
| Exercise guide | 55 |
| **Exercise Programme** | **73** |
| Low back stretches | 74 |
| Low back strengthening | |
|     Level 1 | 83 |
|     Level 2 | 92 |
| Buttock and leg stretches | 97 |
| Neck exercises | 104 |
|     Neck stretching exercises | 105 |
|     Neck strengthening exercises | 109 |
| General Aerobic Exercise Programme | 111 |
| My Action Plan | 118 |
| Exercise Glossary | 122 |
| About the Author | 124 |
| Bibliography | 125 |
| Goals | 126 |
| Testimonials | 128 |

# INTRODUCTION

“ If history tells us anything, it's that knowledge is always evolving, so what we know today is certain to become obsolete or inadequate by tomorrow. Unfortunately, the practice and application of knew knowledge takes time to catch up, and nowhere is this truer than in healthcare. Seeing Nick work with leading edge concepts in back pain medicine is a real breath of fresh air. ”

Dr Adam Al-Kashi
*Head of Research at BackCare – The UK's National Back Pain Association*

# INTRODUCTION

As you may know from your own painful experience, it's not easy to determine the most effective treatment for your back pain. Differing opinions and information surrounding back pain create confusion and doubt in our minds. This overload of information has led to uncertainty about the best path to treating back pain.

Personal Health Plans (PHP) are a way of empowering people with long- term back pain to be able to take greater ownership and responsibility for the condition, which often results in less pain, greater flexibility, and a gradual return to the pre-condition "heaven" that sufferers crave. Over time, we have all become too reliant on the medical profession to treat back pain when, in most cases, the best and most powerful solutions can be provided by us, the sufferers.

A Personal Health Plan can best be described as a focused, determined, and self-help journey over time that manages and controls the condition, builds a stronger body and mind, thereby reducing or even eradicating the pain. Because you and your commitment to achieve a solution primarily drive it, a PHP is often the most beneficial course of treatment to the back pain sufferer and the most cost-effective.

Once you have the knowledge and skills contained in this programme, you can implement it on your own or working in conjunction with both professionals and non-professionals, particularly family and friends. Having additional people involved provides you with a mentoring facility much the same as a Personal Trainer in a gymnasium.

Think of this programme as your road map to the life you want to live. A life where everyday stuff is easier to do, like putting your socks on in the morning, picking up something from the floor, or putting the kids in the car. It may be the life that you have wanted to live for a long time.

# INTRODUCTION

The goal of this programme is to get you started in the right direction. The philosophy behind it is based on the premise that your pain can be affected by both your mind and your body. This programme will give you a solid foundation of knowledge and back pain relieving exercises. By committing to this simple exercise programme, you'll establish healthy new habits that you can build on throughout your life.

A properly structured PHP will help you to:

- A new understanding of how our spine and body works
- Develop a greater understanding of the causes of pain,
- Fully consider your own needs and wishes,
- Provide you with a range of skills to improve the condition,
- Reduce your pain,
- Improve your general health and most importantly,
- Improve your quality of life.

## How is a personal health plan designed?

This programme was written for everyone who is struggling with neck and back pain in their everyday life, and for people who have tried all sorts of treatments or medications and yet have seen no lasting results, or worse yet, have experienced a steady increase in their pain and decline in their everyday function.

The Personal Health Plan is owned and designed by individual sufferers. It is up to each person to decide what information and skills he/she wishes to include in his/her Personal Health Plan.

# INTRODUCTION

The PHP establishes short, medium and long-term goals, and when used properly with personal commitment, the Personal Health Plan will deliver the knowledge and skills for long-term relief.

The PHP has been designed to be flexible, so you can work through it at your own pace in order to allow it to fit in with your life style. You can choose which sections provide the most benefit to support the management of your condition. It can also be used in conjunction with treatment from a healthcare professional. Some people will be happy to complete the Personal Health Plan on their own whilst others will require assistance. If you need help filling in your Personal Health Plan you may want to ask a family member or friend to help you.

Based on current medical research, the PHP offers practical advice and information to help you better control your back pain and make the most of life.

Remember, following a written Back Pain PHP that's been developed especially for you can significantly reduce the long-term effects of back pain. The plan may also need adjusting and updating over time.

## What are the alternatives?

Whilst there is no cure for chronic back pain, there are many ways to manage the pain and reduce or even eradicate the impact it has on your life. A combination of advice, medication, physical exercise, therapies, and a positive mind-set can help you deal with back pain effectively. A Back Pain Personal Health Plan can help you stay on track and manage your back pain so that your health and lifestyle will benefit.

# INTRODUCTION

## Back pain explained

Back pain will affect up to 80% of us in our lifetime. Often there is no obvious cause; however, we do know how to manage and control many of its effects, which is what the Back Pain PHP is all about. In this programme you will find some suggested steps you can take to help lower the risk of back pain, reduce the number of recurrences, and limit the pain caused by it.

There are two main types of back pain:

1. Acute or short-term back pain is the common type and it usually resolves itself in three days to six weeks, whether or not you receive treatment.
2. Chronic back pain exists if pain and symptoms persist for longer than three months. It's useful to know when to seek medical help and that self-care alone will probably not work for you. If you're still unsure after following the programme, a healthcare professional can make that assessment and guide you through your treatment and recovery.

## What you'll learn from this programme

After reading this book, you will have learned:

- How to break the fear and anxiety cycle that keeps you in a vulnerable and painful state.
- A new understanding of how our spine and body works.
- How to increase your confidence levels through exercise.
- How to identify muscular tightness and imbalances.

# INTRODUCTION

- Ways to improve your posture.
- Ways to use stretching to ease the build-up of tense muscles.
- How to gradually strengthen your back muscles as you continue to gain confidence and regain your full range of activity.

The best course of action is to read through the programme so that you can fully comprehend how the information relates to you and your pain. This will increase your understanding and confidence in your back before you start the exercise programme.

The purpose of this programme is to help you to increase your knowledge and understanding of your pain. This is not an instant fix to your pain, but a long, steady road to recovery.

A quick browse through the programme and a couple of days of doing a few exercises isn't going to make much of a dent in the many processes that have caused your pain. I say this not to scare you, but to make sure you understand that it will take time and effort to achieve results.

If you are starting this programme, you are probably in a negative mindset that includes:

- Being scared and confused about what is causing your pain.
- Not knowing how to help ease your pain.
- Being confused about which exercises are best to ease and prevent pain.
- Lacking motivation and the "get up and go" to do something about your pain.

# INTRODUCTION

How do you move away from this negative mindset to embrace a strong, healthy outlook? Here are strategies to help you get and stay motivated.

## Strategy 1: set goals

Your motivation should be directly linked to a plan of action. If you're not clear on where you are going and how you are going to get there, you're setting yourself up for a fall.

Your goals should be specific and measurable. For example, let's say that in a specified period of time you want to be able to walk for thirty minutes, be able to play football with the kids, or even to be able to put your socks on in the morning.

For best results establish short, intermediate and long-term goals. Here are some examples of each:

**Short-Term Goal:** "I want to establish a back exercise regime, slowly increasing my repetitions to ten over the next month."

**Intermediate Goal:** "In three months, I want to be able to walk the kids to school and vacuum the house."

**Long-Term Goal:** "In six months' time, I want to be able to go back to my old class in the gym."

# INTRODUCTION

To achieve these objectives, set yourself **daily goals.** You must take specific actions that are in line with your longer-range objectives.

Each day, set yourself a plan:

- Know which exercises and how many repetitions you are going to do.
- Plan how many minutes of aerobic exercise you will do that day.
- Don't forget to congratulate yourself and be proud of your achievements when you complete your daily or weekly goals.
- Discipline yourself to keep a back exercise journal.

Remember, you wouldn't be reading this if you didn't want to get back to the life you want!

## Strategy 2: remain focused

At first, your body will want to resist the changes you are going to make. It's the body's natural urge to maintain the status quo by raising physical defences to unfamiliar physical exertion. For the first few days, your muscles and joints will feel tight and sore. Remember that the exercise programme is designed to progress at a slow, gradual pace.

# INTRODUCTION

## Strategy 3: form partnerships

If you know someone who experiences similar pain and problems to yourself, such as a friend, work colleague of even your partner, encourage them to join you in reading this programme, setting goals, and going through the back exercise programme together. Having someone to share the experience with you can help keep you both on the right track.

## Strategy 4: accept setbacks

During your path to recovery, you may have the odd bad day when you really ache. Accept this as part of the process, pace your activities that day and resume the programme as soon as possible. The longer you stick with the programme, the fewer setbacks you will experience.

Before you begin working towards your goals, you need to be in the right state of mind. In Part One of this programme, we'll explore the powerful role your mind plays in helping you recover from the physical manifestations of back pain.

During the programme you will be asked questions about your health, your future goals, and how you want to achieve these goals. It is important you partake in each section in order to plan a structured route to your recovery.

You will now be asked to complete the About Me section. This will help you identify areas of your health that could be improved.

### Let's get started!

# ABOUT ME

The About Me section will help you identify areas of your health that could be improved. All you have to do is answer these simple questions.

| **What it might help others to know about me.** |
|---|
| For example, record details of personality, likes, and dislikes. |

| **Where is your pain and when do you suffer most from it?** |
|---|
| For example, the pain is in my low back especially when I sit for a while. |

| **These are the concerns I have about my back pain and wellbeing:** |
|---|
| Consider psychological, emotional, and social as well as physical issues. |

| **These are the areas of my current health and wellbeing that could be improved:** |
|---|
| Consider diet, exercise, and lifestyle. |

| **These are my main health and wellbeing needs:** |
|---|
| These are the main priorities for my current and future health. |

The Back Pain PHP will teach you skills in order to improve and cope better with your pain. As you go through the programme note down in your Action Plan, which can be found on page 118, the skills or knowledge you have learnt, and then how you will put this into action in order to achieve your goals.

# CHANGING YOUR MIND

> " This is an important book. Bringing together leading-edge insights from the field of mind-body healing with his own experience as a physiotherapist Nick Sinfield offers a comprehensive guide book to recovering from back pain. You are in safe hands. "

*Dr Mark Atkinson,*
*medical doctor, founder of the Academy of Human Potential*
*and author of "The Mind-Body Bible"*

# CHANGING YOUR MIND

Back pain continues to increase throughout the Western world. Whether it affects the neck, shoulders, low back, or upper buttock area, it can have a crippling effect on every aspect of a person's life. It can affect their ability to work and earn a living, enjoy recreational activities, and participate fully in life. And it can affect their emotional and mental wellbeing, leaving them fearful, frustrated, and hopeless.

## Modern medicine: improved diagnostics, worsening outcomes

Why has the prevalence of back pain continued to rise, even as modern diagnostic and treatment options become more and more sophisticated and widely available? Magnetic resonance imaging (MRI), computer tomography (CT), and X-rays allow doctors to see our muscles, nerves, bones, and spinal canal, and accurately pinpoint abnormalities that can cause pain. Every hidden element of our physical condition can be mapped and analysed, yet many of us continue to be plagued by pain and immobility.

Why isn't modern medicine able to help?

The answer may lie in the fact that modern medicine focuses on the physical dimensions of back pain. Elaborate diagnostic equipment is designed to lay bare the innermost workings of the human body and uncover structural abnormalities in the spine. Many prescribed treatments are then based on addressing those abnormalities.

The diagnostic and treatment cycle deals substantially with the physical manifestations of the condition.

# CHANGING YOUR MIND

Yet recent medical research demonstrates the positive effects of psychological interventions, such as Cognitive Behavioral Therapy for the treatment of chronic low back pain.

It's no wonder that so many back pain patients experience unpredictable treatment outcomes! And it's no wonder that doctors and their patients have become so pessimistic about the possibility of long-term success in treating back pain.

## Treating the mind and body

The idea that a physical condition can also have a psychological component is difficult for some people to believe. But as our pain becomes ingrained in our minds and bodies, our perception of the pain changes along with our behaviour towards it. These changes in our minds and bodies can create a chronic pain cycle. Emotional tension also has a proven ability to induce physiological change, including soft tissue changes that express itself as muscular tension and simple back strains.

In the same way that emotional stress can suppress our immune systems and affect our resilience to disease, it can have a detrimental impact on our soft tissue structures.

## Knowledge is the key to recovery

Successful and permanent treatment for back pain must be based on educating back pain sufferers. This is accomplished by teaching them to recognise and change ingrained perceptions and beliefs in their pain and the resulting emotional stress this produces. This holistic approach, which treats back pain as a physical, mental, and emotional issue, offers a more effective and lasting

# CHANGING YOUR MIND

treatment option. By training the pain sufferer to recognise and change their perceptions and beliefs, we are able to add a powerful psychological dimension to existing, physically based treatment options.

This programme is designed to educate the reader about back pain and provide a clear set of guidelines for healing back pain and changing your behaviour towards it. As you read, you will learn to recognise how your own pain has created a damaging behavioural pattern. You'll also learn to use simple techniques to change these behaviours before they can affect your physical condition. You'll gradually be able to master these psychological techniques and recognise how your pain can be improved through self-management strategies.

With the techniques you learn in this programme, you are going to take back control from your back pain!

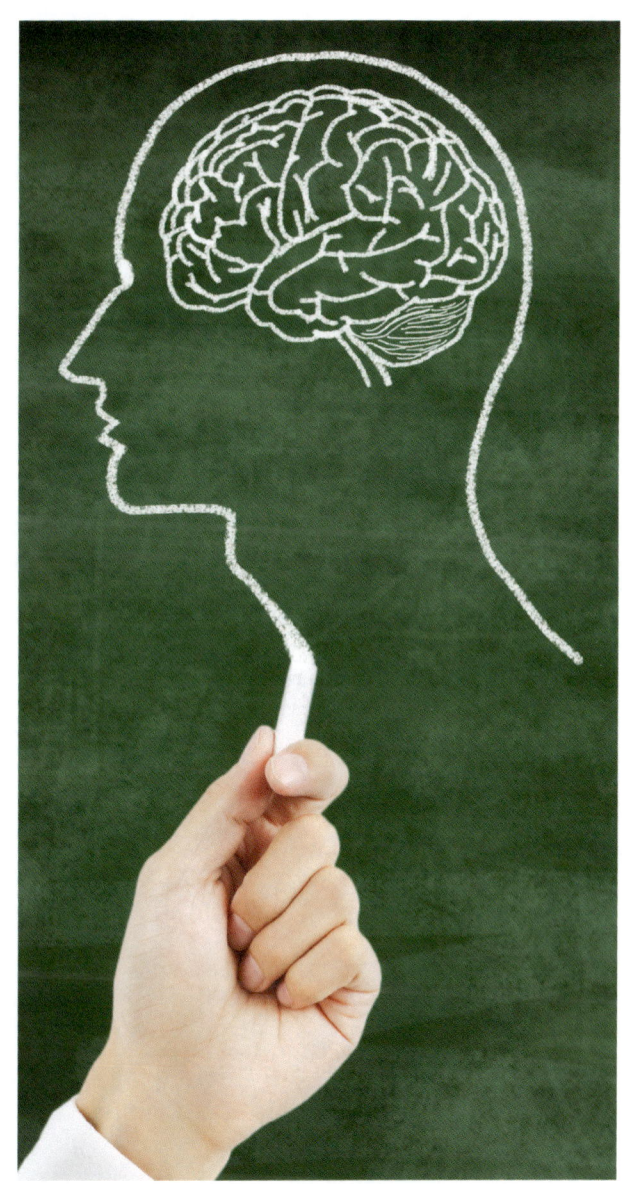

# CHANGING YOUR MIND

You'll learn:

- Why X-rays and MRI results may not correlate to patient symptoms.
- Why you are the best person to control your recovery.
- How to overcome fear and vulnerability.
- How to learn to "trust" your back again.
- How to actively plan your recovery and guard against recurrence.
- Clear and easy to understand back exercises.

Plus you'll get a step-by-step guide to self-managing your back pain.

So read on, keep an open mind and be prepared to learn something new about your health!

## Understanding pain

Injury and structural issues, such as a simple strained muscle or inflammatory responses to structural problems in the spine, can cause acute back pain. This should settle in time as the healing process takes place. Therefore why can pain persist after tissues have had plenty of time to heal?

Pain is a multidimensional and complicated experience for the sufferer, with many contributing and interacting mechanisms. These mechanisms can be a mixture of contributory elements comprising emotional and physical causes, and with a better understanding of pain you will be better equipped to find your route to recovery.

# CHANGING YOUR MIND

Your nervous system, which produces pain, is highly adaptable to change. Triggers such as injury or stress can result in an increased concentration of neural impulses from inflamed, scarred, weak, or acidic tissues around the spinal cord. This increases the sensitivity within the nervous system, meaning more pain signals transferred to the brain. If this continues over time these sensory distortions can cause things to hurt that didn't hurt before and a loss of ability to activate muscles that help stabilise the spine.

This means that simply touching the skin, or a cold breeze, might cause pain signals to be sent to the brain.

This enhanced sensitivity of the nervous system is nearly always a main feature in persistent pain. Remember that the pain is normal, not harmful. Your brain is being tricked to protect you.

## Understand and overcome

If you're not given an answer to the cause of your pain, it's easy to become worried, confused, and anxious. This in turn may cause more tightness in the soft tissues around the back and neck, especially if you concentrate on the pain. This can cause ongoing back pain.

This can be described as Tension Related Pain (TRP) a very common symptom with chronic back pain sufferers. It can affect us all differently; for some it will be the main cause of pain and to others a smaller influence.

# CHANGING YOUR MIND

As you progress through the programme you will learn to identify if TRP is one of the causes or the main cause to your pain. This will change your mindset, help to ease your anxiety and confusion to the cause of the pain, and allow you to move onto the exercise programme with confidence.

The latest medical research demonstrates a need for an integrated mind and body treatment programme for back pain. As you learn and understand more about your pain through this programme, it will become obvious what changes are required to improve your pain through goal setting.

## Looking forwards not backwards

Negative past experiences related to your back pain, such as a discussion with a healthcare professional, can create negative self-beliefs. This can affect your present life in unhealthy and unhelpful ways. If you think in a negative way towards your back, this can produce negative feelings and lead to pain in these areas. These negative thoughts or feelings relating to your back pain will produce negative actions and behaviours in relation to your pain, causing a vicious cycle of pain.

## Your thoughts and feelings produce your actions

You may benefit from working on changing these thoughts to be more realistic rather than thinking the worst. If you imagine the worst, this may become reality, as your thoughts produce feelings and behaviours.

# CHANGING YOUR MIND

> **Write down any specific events that could have led to your current feelings relating to your back pain.**
>
> 

> **Now write down how your back makes you feel. Here are a few suggestions: anxious, stressed, sad, hopeless, guilty, frustrated, angry, or confused.**
>
> 

Now begin to understand how it will be helpful to change your feelings to these past experiences in order to move forwards.

Recognise these feelings because they will cause you to currently behave in certain ways to cope with your back pain. This may help in the short term but may hinder your long term recovery

The experiences and suffering you have had in the past with your back do not mean the future will be the same.

## Think healthy!

# CHANGING YOUR MIND

## Risks and benefits

Developing new feelings and thoughts around your back pain, such as starting to exercise again, can feel unnatural and risky. It will require practise and perseverance to build these thoughts into action. It is important to keep learning about new forms of exercise and knowledge about back rehabilitation to reinforce your new feelings.

If your past actions and behaviours have failed to improve your pain, what have you got to lose by trying something new?

Change unhelpful thoughts from "My back will never get better" to "I am going to focus on an exercise programme to help me improve my quality of life."

This programme will take time and effort, so set yourself mini goals to reach your long term goals. Even walking one minute further every week will add up before you know it.

Remember your health is a work in progress. Every skill or new piece of knowledge will provide you with the ability to change, adapt and develop in order to reach your goals.

In order to reach your goals you need to accept personal responsibility to improve your health. This self-acceptance will allow you to take the next steps on your journey to recovery.

If you avoid tasks or movements because you think it will flare up your pain, you may have negative coping strategies and avoid certain tasks or exercises, which lead to building fear. This can lead to overestimating the damage these tasks will cause and underestimate how much you can do and how strong your back is.

# CHANGING YOUR MIND

It may not be as bad or as difficult as you expected!

Do not give yourself any excuses. Buy the right clothing, footwear, or an exercise mat, and commit to your recovery.

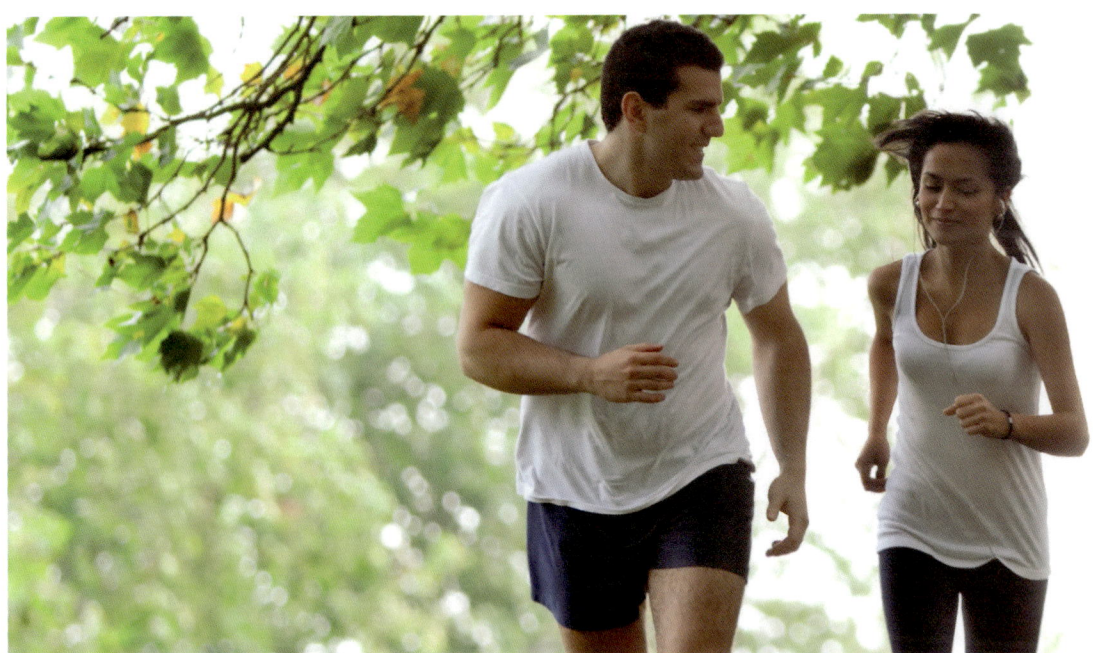

 Think differently! No excuses – get moving! Your back is made to move, bend, and twist.

# CHANGING YOUR MIND

## Exercise

**Describe how your pain has made you feel or behave, and how this has effected your actions. For example: I don't do any back exercises because they hurt too much or housework makes my back ache.**

**Predict what will happen if you try this. For example: My pain is always worse after I do this_____.**

# CHANGING YOUR MIND

Now try it – what have you got to lose? You can always go back to what you used to do.

| What were the results? |
| --- |
|   |

## Concentration and mindfulness

A basic definition of mindfulness is to accept who we are and what we are experiencing in any given moment. Use this level of focus to connect with your body right now. Connect with your muscles – how they tense then relax; and your joints – how they move and bend. This technique can be used to revert your attention to this away from your pain. Force your attention away from the pain to the exercise you are performing.

# CHANGING YOUR MIND

In this introduction to mindfulness we will learn to accept the condition of our spine's health in this present moment and relearn how the deep abdominal breathing muscles function.

Mindfulness is an effective way to manage our anxiety and negative thoughts towards our back pain. This exercise gives us the chance to connect with our bodies through breathing and concentration.

This exercise will require your full attention, through deep concentration, on your present breath and how your respiratory muscles achieve this.

During the exercise you may feel your mind drift off. When this happens, bring your mind back to focus on the task. Remember this will take practice so be patient!

Start with five minutes a day and you soon find that you will be able to focus your attention for longer.

## Mindfulness breathing exercise

- Start off lying on your back with your knees bent and your feet on the floor. Support your head with a pillow if needed.
- Place your hands on your stomach and notice how your breath feels in this moment.

# CHANGING YOUR MIND

- Imagine you have a balloon in your stomach, which inflates and deflates with each in- and out-breath. Focus on your stomach rising with the in-breath and falling with the out-breath. Keep your awareness present with the breath.
- As your mind wanders keep pulling your thoughts back to your breath, then refocus your attention to the present moment. Concentrate on how this creates a feeling of calmness. Do not allow yourself to be distracted by thoughts, feelings, or sounds.

After two weeks you can expect to see improvements in your overall wellbeing and stress levels. This mindfulness exercise can be transferred to many other exercises in order to connect with your body and accept imbalances or limitations. Through this acceptance you will be able to focus positively on how to improve your pain.

**Keep it simple!**
- If an area of your back feels stiff, stretch it!
- If your back feels weak, strengthen it!

## The vicious cycle of diagnosis, fear, and recurrence

Many of us are used to perceiving our backs as weak and easily damaged, and we subsequently begin to worry and grow fearful. You may even become anxious about hurting your back further. You become despondent about your

# CHANGING YOUR MIND

poor health and concerned about your future. This accumulation of anxiety and stress, in turn, can cause a change in your behaviour towards exercising and how you use your back in everyday life. And it is these changes that can cause your back pain to flare up and recur again and again.

Now ask yourself if you're locked in a vicious cycle of diagnosis, fear about the diagnosis, and a recurrence caused by the psychological stress of your pain and your ensuing changes in behaviour.

Modern medical investigations can evoke a fearful reaction that, in turn, prolongs and worsens your pain. It is very important for you to be able to recognise and address any resulting behavioural changes that may have taken place. By seeking a cure for your pain, you have in fact only generated more worry and anxiety in your condition.

## Why has the incidence of back pain increased rapidly over the past thirty years?

One answer could be the number of patients being diagnosed with structural abnormalities. More and more people are being scanned, X-rayed, and then told, "There's something wrong." As a result, more and more people are succumbing to anxiety about their condition, and that anxiety could create an increase of TRP.

The reality is that these physical abnormalities were prevalent long before MRIs and other diagnostic tools were invented.

Most of us have structural abnormalities in our backs. Everyone's back is different and develops in different ways as we grow and age. Everyone's back has been subjected to the stress of physical activity, trauma, health changes,

# CHANGING YOUR MIND

and other effects. But those structural abnormalities don't necessarily cause back pain. It's very important for back pain sufferers to understand that almost all spinal abnormalities are the normal effects of ageing.

Here are some examples:
**Degenerative discs:** Our discs often accumulate wear and tear, especially in the low back region. It's a perfectly normal (and harmless) part of the aging process, and an inevitable effect of gravity.

**Low back, neck, and shoulder blade pain:** Recurring pain is most common in these areas. Revealingly, these areas are also the most likely to be the site of soft tissue dysfunction caused by tightness or weakness of the surrounding muscles and other soft tissue structures.

**Nerve related symptoms:** The sharp burning, tingling or numbness that accompanies nerve damage can be terrifying for the affected patient, but it is often caused by pressure placed on the affected nerves by inflammation following an injury.

In short, it may not be the structural abnormalities that are causing pain.

People often misdiagnose themselves or accept a medical diagnosis that attributes their back pain to a structural abnormality that will lead to a lifetime of pain. This can lead to a change in behaviour. Alternatively, people believe that their pain is a result of a degenerative process, an abnormality, or general weakness. And of course, the prevalence of physical diagnostic equipment only feeds into that prejudice.

**Let's take a look at this "vicious cycle" of pain:**

# CHANGING YOUR MIND

## The Vicious Cycle of Pain

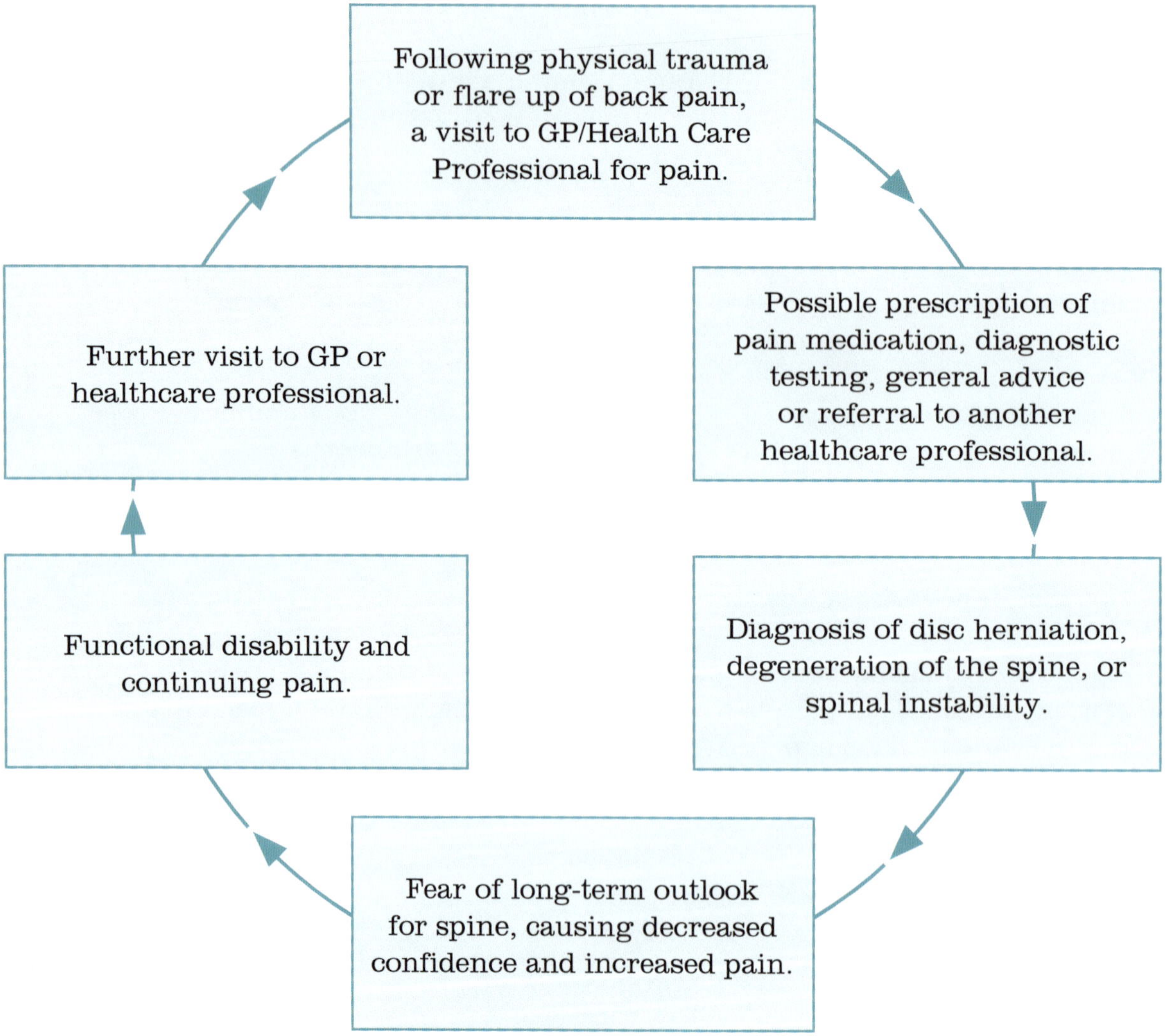

- Following physical trauma or flare up of back pain, a visit to GP/Health Care Professional for pain.
- Possible prescription of pain medication, diagnostic testing, general advice or referral to another healthcare professional.
- Diagnosis of disc herniation, degeneration of the spine, or spinal instability.
- Fear of long-term outlook for spine, causing decreased confidence and increased pain.
- Functional disability and continuing pain.
- Further visit to GP or healthcare professional.

# CHANGING YOUR MIND

## Recognising tension related pain

So, how can we recognise TRP and assess its impact on our back health and related pain levels? We can start by acknowledging sources of stress and tension in our lives.

Stress and tension can come from a number of areas of our life:

- Family conflicts and responsibilities.
- Too much work and not enough support in the work environment.
- Financial problems, debt and worries about the future.
- Unresolved childhood issues of anger or low self-esteem.
- Unrealistically high expectations for ourselves.

If you can relate to any of these scenarios, there's a good chance that you carry some level of harmful stress and tension in your body. This emotional stress can then express itself as painful physical tension. This type of pain is most likely to show up in certain areas, including:

- Neck, top of shoulders and shoulder blades.
- The lower back area.
- Outer aspects of the buttocks.

Tellingly, these are also areas that medical professionals identify as being most likely to be deprived of oxygen due to constricting muscular tightness, which is the kind of contraction that occurs with tension and emotional stress.

# CHANGING YOUR MIND

Although these areas are very common sites of emotionally triggered pain, TRP can occur in other areas, and can also move around through the network of muscles, bones and nerves. Often, patients with TRP report pain that migrates to a new location as the old location starts to improve.

## How do we stop the cycle of pain?

If conventional medical diagnosis and treatment is unsuccessful to cure your back pain, what methods can you use to stop the cycle of pain?

The first step in treating your pain effectively may be to recognise the psychological elements of your condition and any resulting behavioural changes. Until you are willing to accept the role your actions and behaviours play in your back pain, you'll struggle to improve. You'll continue to be caught up in the vicious cycle of conventional diagnosis, fear, stress, and pain. Once you are ready to acknowledge that your physical pain may have a behavioural pattern, you'll be able to open yourself up to a conscious programme that involves training yourself to recognise those damaging feelings. You'll be able to:

1. Stop worrying about your pain.
2. Recognise your pre-programmed "pain patterns."
3. Acknowledge and deal with your feelings.
4. Resist the urge to fall back on "physical" diagnoses.

Let's take a closer look at each of these important steps.

# CHANGING YOUR MIND

## 1. Stop worrying about your pain

After being incapacitated by back pain, it's hard not to worry when you feel a twinge. Even people who have never experienced back pain before are likely to react with fear after being told that back pain is caused by a degenerative process. It's easy to react to the onset of back pain by imagining the worst that can happen – a degenerative condition, reduced mobility, missed work, and weeks or months of pain.

However, it's important to resist the urge to wallow in fear and anxiety. The best thing you can do for your health is to overcome your apprehension, keep moving, and return to your normal activities.

## 2. Recognise your pre-pregrammed "pain patterns"

Did you know that you actively programme or condition your body to experience pain? By simply anticipating that a particular activity or situation will cause pain, you set up a pain pathway in your brain. For instance, you may assume that the act of getting in the car and driving is likely to cause a back flare-up – and sure enough, the next time you get into your car, you feel a twinge. Or perhaps you associate bending forwards or lifting things with back pain. You may have sustained a back injury whilst engaged in a particular activity, such as playing a sport. It's likely that whenever you play that sport in future, you hold anxiety about the possibility of a re-occurrence of back pain. These associations between a particular activity and the likelihood of pain are called "pain patterns," and they can actually cause you to bring on back pain through anxiety and stress.

# CHANGING YOUR MIND

## 3. Acknowledge and deal with your emotions

To deal with the impact of emotions on your physical health, you need to be honest about those emotions. If you are a worrier or a "type A" personality, overly responsible at home or at work, compulsive and a perfectionist, you need to acknowledge those traits in yourself. People most likely to suffer from TRP are often competitive, ambitious, goal-oriented and deeply driven to succeed. They put an intense pressure on themselves, which can lead to stress and anxiety.

Gaining an awareness of your psychological type and your tendency to internalise stress is critical in managing those pressures and controlling their effect on your back health. Think about how you deal with feelings of anger and anxiety. Sometimes, you may not even be aware that you hold those emotional tensions in your body, because they exist at the subconscious level. But it is helpful to ask yourself, "How do I deal with my emotions?"

For instance, try to be honest about how you deal with your anger. Do you tend to address it directly and try to resolve the issue? Or do you repress it and then release it at inappropriate times? If you hold repressed anger, you might have incidences of road rage in your past, or have a tendency to "snap" over small irritations.

The same is true of sadness, frustration, disappointment and a host of other negative emotions. If we don't handle our feelings in healthy ways, they create tension in the body; this tension can express itself as muscular pain. This pain, in turn, serves to distract attention away from the emotional realm and towards the physical realm. In this way, people subconsciously avoid dealing with their feelings, and instead expend their energies on coping with a physical complaint. Unfortunately, this means that they are unlikely to resolve their physical pain, as the emotional tension will surface again and again until it is addressed.

# CHANGING YOUR MIND

## 4. Resist the urge to fall back on "physical" diagnoses

Today's medical profession is increasingly able to use diagnostic tools such as MRI, CT scans, and X-rays to diagnose structural dysfunctions of the spine. But these methods can also interpret perfectly normal, degenerative changes in our spine as abnormal and painful conditions. These diagnoses, in turn, create fears and anxieties that make us treat our backs as fragile, delicate structures that are prone to damage and require endless instructions on how to sit, stand, bend, work and lift.

Moreover these conventional diagnoses that identify physical degeneration as the source of their pain are very convincing. X-rays and scans seem so impressive to the patient that it seems impossible that the pain could be caused by anything else. What this means is that it's all too easy to accept that either you

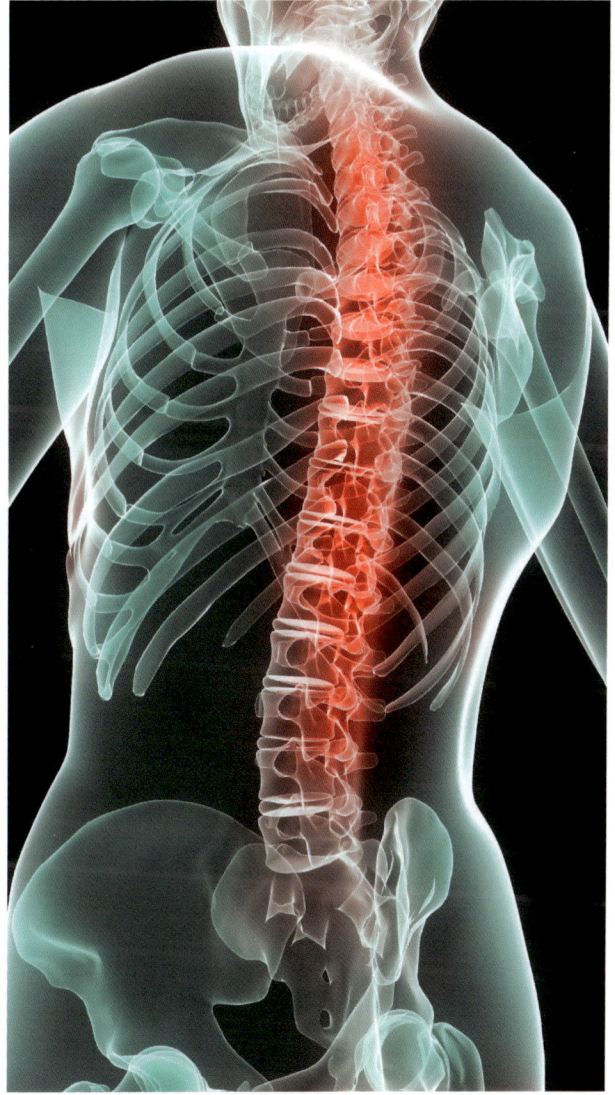

# CHANGING YOUR MIND

will need surgery or you will have back pain for the rest of your life. But it's important that you keep an open mind and fully explore how you are going to self manage your recovery.

Nearly a century ago, the groundbreaking neurologist Sigmund Freud said that many physical ailments had their basis in emotional tensions. Today, in the face of increasing evidence, medical science is finally starting to accept the central role our emotions play in our overall health. New research is emerging about the interrelation between our minds and bodies. Science is only just beginning to untangle the ways in which the two affect one another, but the fact remains that they do, and you can use this knowledge to make a positive change in your quality of life!

**Let's take a closer look at the relationship between emotional stress, behavioural changes and pain.**

# CHANGING YOUR MIND

## The Relationship Between Stress and Pain

- Our repressed emotions/feelings (anxiety/stress/anger/sadness/frustration/etc.) exist in our subconscious mind.
- When emotions are not consciously addressed and resolved, they transfer to the body because they have nowhere else to go.
- The emotional stress causes the autonomic nervous system (an involuntary system in the body controlling the blood flow to our tissues) to restrict blood and oxygen to our muscles and nerves.
- Muscles deprived of oxygen begin to build up deposits of lactic acid (waste chemicals).
- Affected muscles and the surrounding nerves cause pain, spasm, tingling, or numbness.
- Our conscious brain now chooses to concentrate on our physical pain, NOT our repressed emotional feelings.

# CHANGING YOUR MIND

So how do we prevent the formation of TRP in the muscles and soft tissues surrounding our spine?

Here's how:

We need to commit to a treatment programme that allows us to understand TRP, accept its role in our health and how our feelings and behaviours contribute to the pain, and then use a combination of psychological and physical techniques to resolve our pain once and for all.

Let's take a more detailed look at the four stages involved in the recovery programme.

## The four step recovery programme

### Stage 1. Education and understanding
- Learn how your feelings and behaviours are contributing to your pain.
- Learn how TRP can affect the human body and cause pain.

### Stage 2. Acceptance of current negative behaviours and increased confidence of recovery
- Recognise the cycle of pain/diagnosis/fear/more pain.
- Accept that you are the best person to self-manage your back pain.

### Stage 3. Integration of new understanding into daily life
- Use exercise to stimulate blood flow and oxygen to areas of pain.
- Start to return to previous activities with confidence.
- Regain confidence and knowledge of how your body works and any imbalances in the muscles.

# CHANGING YOUR MIND

### Stage 4. Ongoing recovery and prevention
- Use awareness, acceptance and exercise integration together for the long-term resolution of your pain.

Through these treatment stages, this programme approaches your back pain in a holistic manner, with both mind and body engaged throughout. The mind/body approach includes:

**1. Knowledge therapy:** Educating yourself about the self-management of back pain and fully accepting that your behaviours can affect your physicality. Gaining awareness of your behavioural patterns and re-programming your responses.

**2. Exercise therapy:** Building confidence, strengthening your spine, and returning to full functionality and health.

Your treatment success will depend on your ability to maintain an open mind, a strong awareness of the ways in which mind and body interact, and a willingness to address and change your patterns of thought and behaviour.

It may take time to be able to get beyond the immediacy of the pain and see deeper into which behaviours require changing. Your mind is a very sophisticated machine, and it will not be easy to resist the tricks it can play on you. However, each time you make an effort to change a behavioural pattern, you will be subtly shifting your brain patterns and making it easier, each time, to forge new pathways to easing the source of your back pain.

# CHANGING YOUR MIND

### Tell your mind that you are in charge!
Each day, commit to making a conscious effort to see through the tricks your mind can play on you. Focus on your thoughts and feelings and the tension it creates in your body, rather than the specific area of pain. Remind yourself on a daily basis that you are actively engaged in a process of taking charge of your health and changing your behavioural patterns towards the pain.

### Tell your body to get moving!
As you develop a new awareness of how your thoughts and feelings produce your actions:

- Begin to lose that familiar sense of fear about the condition of your back.
- Stop feeling as through your spine is fragile and can be harmed by a single wrong move.
- Start to feel stronger and more confident about moving naturally and freely.

Instead of keeping yourself in a fear-based state of inactivity, get up, move around, and embrace a full and physically active life.

Once you start to change your feelings towards your back pain, your recovery may be gradual but steady. As you gain strength and confidence, you will begin to enjoy your exercise programme and see positive results.

By consciously fostering a hopeful attitude and a positive mental outlook, you can learn to self manage your back pain recovery. This is a proven therapeutic process, so give your health the attention and commitment it deserves.

Can you imagine yourself healing your back through an integrated mental/physical programme?

# PREVENTION AND TREATMENT

*❝ This is a fantastic book. It is very informative, and offers clear and sensible guidance to help patients manage their low back pain. ❞*

*James Langdon*
*BSc(Hons) MBBS(Eng) FRCS(Ortho),*
*Consultant Orthopaedic Spinal Surgeon,*
*West Hertfordshire Hospitals NHS Trust*

# PREVENTION AND TREATMENT

Your back is involved in almost every movement you make and is in action whether you are walking, standing, lying, sitting, balancing, or holding your posture or your position. Our spines have evolved to bend, twist and rotate to take us through life!

Your spine is comprised of twenty-five bones called vertebrae, stacked on top of each other, resting on the pelvis (your hips) and topped by the skull. Between each pair of vertebrae is a tough, spongy cushion called a disc. These discs act as shock absorbers as well as providing for movement of each vertebra in relation to the next, giving the spine flexibility, allowing us to move through everyday life.

Strong ligaments and muscles hold the vertebrae and discs firmly together in a column called the spinal column. The spine also provides a protective case for the spinal cord that runs from the brain, by way of a canal through the middle of the vertebrae down to the lower back. The spinal cord forms the main communication channel between the brain and the rest of the body via the nerves that branch off at intervals through spaces between the vertebrae.

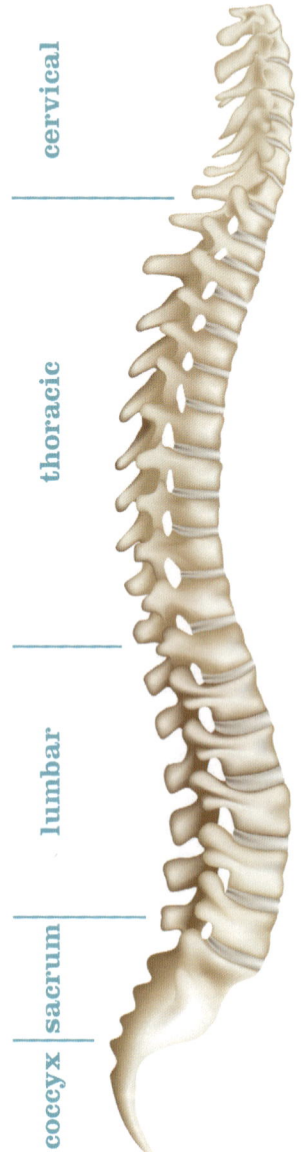

# PREVENTION AND TREATMENT

## Causes of back pain

Most back pain is called "simple mechanical back pain" and is caused by strains and minor injury, or simply not looking after our bodies during our everyday life.

Although the pain comes on quickly and can be triggered by a particular movement, the cause may have been building up for some time. A specific diagnosis may not be necessary in order to treat and manage simple back pain effectively.

It is important to note that people without any symptoms of back pain can also have findings on X-ray such as osteoarthritis, lumbar spondylosis (degeneration of the lower spine), and degenerative discs. Therefore the findings can be inconclusive as they may show other problems but not the cause of the actual pain. Finding the perfect spine would be quite a challenge!

## Treatment for acute back pain

Back pain can have a negative impact on your life. The following advice may help you manage pain and develop a positive approach to your well-being. If your back pain has recently commenced or has suffered a "flare up," there are some measures you can take that may alleviate the pain. These include:

- **Ice and heat:** Try an ice pack for the first 48 to 72 hours. Then use a heat pad.
- **Activity and rest:** In order to reduce inflammation and relieve the symptoms, limit any physical activity that increases the pain. Prolonged periods in bed can cause symptoms to persist and there is evidence that this can be harmful.

# PREVENTION AND TREATMENT

- Avoid any heavy lifting or repetitive twisting to your back until your symptoms settle.
- **Medication:** Anti-inflammatories such as ibuprofen are widely known and used in back pain. These reduce inflammation around the affected areas such as muscles, joints, and ligaments. However, known side effects include gastro-intestinal bleeding, so if you have stomach ulcers or a similar condition these drugs should only be taken under the direction of your doctor. Paracetemol is also effective in pain relief and does not aggravate a stomach condition. Remember that trying to avoid medication can force you to hold yourself stiffly or move in an unnatural way, which creates a cycle of pain, making symptoms worse and prolonging the episode. The medication information outlined here is for general explanatory purposes only and is not medical advice. You should always check with your doctor prior to taking any medication.
- **Sleeping position:** Try sleeping in a curled-up foetal position with a pillow between your legs. If you sleep on your back, place a pillow or rolled towel under your knees to ease the pressure on your spine.
- **Exercise:** Keeping fit is important, so maintain your exercise programme, beginning with light cardiovascular training, walking, or swimming. This will boost the blood flow to your back and promote healing. Stretching and strengthening exercises are also helpful in improving stability and protecting your back in the long term. If you are unsure, your doctor or physiotherapist can help you decide when you should begin exercising.

# PREVENTION AND TREATMENT

## Long term back pain management

Exercise is an essential part of any back pain management programme.

Try to exercise every day, even for a twenty minute session. In your weekly programme include two sessions of mobility and strengthening exercises for key back muscle groups. Also, include some cardiovascular exercises for your heart and lungs. However, don't push your body too far.

If you still feel pain two hours after exercising, it's a signal that you have been doing too much or you may be doing the wrong type of exercise.

With all mobility or stretching exercises, you move your joints as far as they can comfortably go in each direction. The goal is to decrease stiffness and pain while maintaining flexibility and improving joint function.

Cardiovascular exercises are endurance exercises that increase your overall fitness by improving your heart and lung function as well as circulation. The most beneficial exercises are often simply walking, cycling, and swimming. These work to strengthen muscle groups and improve cardiovascular fitness while minimising the impact on your joints.

Develop an exercise programme to increase strength and flexibility in your back muscles and work with them to achieve some daily activity goals. A healthcare professional can also advise you on other physical therapies including heat, ice, massage, acupuncture, and ultrasound, which may also provide supplementary pain relief.

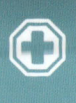

# PREVENTION AND TREATMENT

## Guidelines for back pain prevention

There are ways to avoid damaging your back. Being aware of situations where your back is at risk of injury may help to prevent any damage to your back. The risk of back pain is highest if you are overweight, a smoker or pregnant.

You are also at risk if you do not look after your posture when sitting or standing.

When you lift and carry without the correct posture, you are putting your back at risk.

Being stressed or depressed can also make you vulnerable to pain and injury. You can lessen or perhaps avoid back pain by improving your overall level of fitness and learning how the body works and how to move heavy objects safely.

So take care of your back, don't take risks and follow these guidelines for back pain prevention.

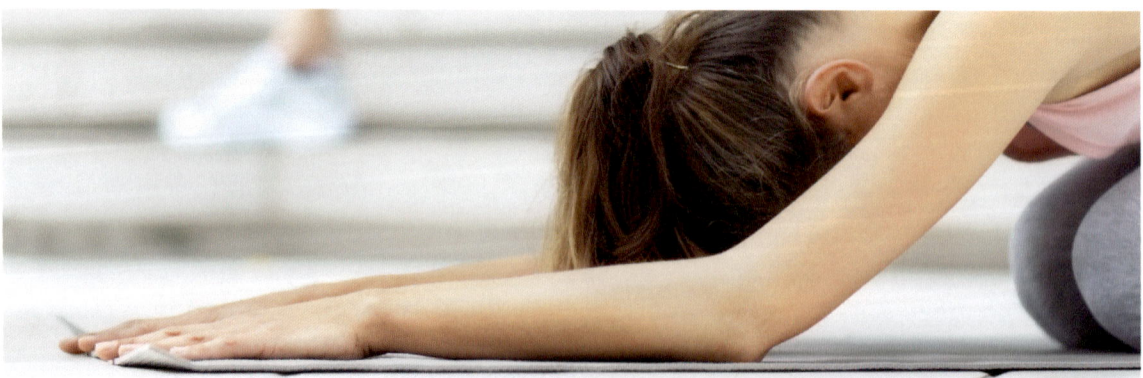

# PREVENTION AND TREATMENT

- Exercise. Regular low-impact aerobic activities that don't strain or jolt your back can increase strength and endurance in your back and allow your muscles to function better. Walking and swimming are good choices. Talk with your physiotherapist about which activities are best for you. It's important to exercise regularly because an inactive lifestyle contributes to lower back pain. Abdominal and back strengthening exercises help condition the muscles so they work together like a natural "corset" for your back.
- Maintain a healthy weight. Being overweight puts strain on your back muscles. If you're overweight, trimming down can reduce your chance of getting back pain.
- Improve your posture during the day. Don't slouch, as poor posture puts a strain on your lower back.
- At night, adjust your sleeping position until you feel comfortable. Choose a firm, supportive mattress with no "valleys."
- Place a small pillow or rolled towel behind your lower back while sitting or driving for long periods of time.
- Avoid wearing high heels, and use cushioned soles when walking.
- Quit smoking, as it is linked to back pain and may reduce pain. It will also lower the risk of heart disease, cancer and other diseases.
- Try practising relaxation techniques such as yoga and tai chi, or have a massage.
- Keep a positive attitude about your job and home life. Studies have shown that people who are unhappy at work or home tend to have more back problems and take longer to recover.

# PREVENTION AND TREATMENT

## Lifting guidelines for back safety

Whether you have chronic back pain or a healthy pain-free back, it is most important to lift heavy objects in a safe and supportive way.

Follow these tips to prevent injury to your back:

### Plan
- Plan what you want to do and don't hurry.
- Separate your feet shoulder-width apart to give you a solid base of support.
- Bend at the knees. Maintain the natural curve of your spine; don't bend at your waist.
- Tighten your stomach muscles.

### Position
- Position the object close to your body before lifting.
- Lift with your legs, not your back. Bend your knees until you are in a squatting position and then straighten at the knees – don't bend at the waist.
- When you need to move heavy objects, push rather than pull.
- When appropriate, use an assistive device such as a transfer belt, sliding board, or draw sheet to move heavy objects or people.

### Avoid
- Avoid trying to lift something that is too heavy or an awkward shape on your own. Seek help.
- Avoid twisting your body. Instead, point your toes in the direction you want to move in and pivot in that direction.

# PREVENTION AND TREATMENT

## Office Ergonomic Advice

Good office ergonomics assists in providing a safe and comfortable work environment. There are a few basics that can help when setting up a work area for computer related tasks. Many of these principles can be transferred to other types of work stations.

Let's talk about posture and try and understand the best way to set up a work station. One of the most important concepts is the idea of a neutral body position. This means that your body's position allows your joints, muscles, connective tissues such as tendons, and the skeletal system to naturally align with minimal effort. The intent of a neutral body position is that it reduces the risk of developing a musculoskeletal disorder (MSD).

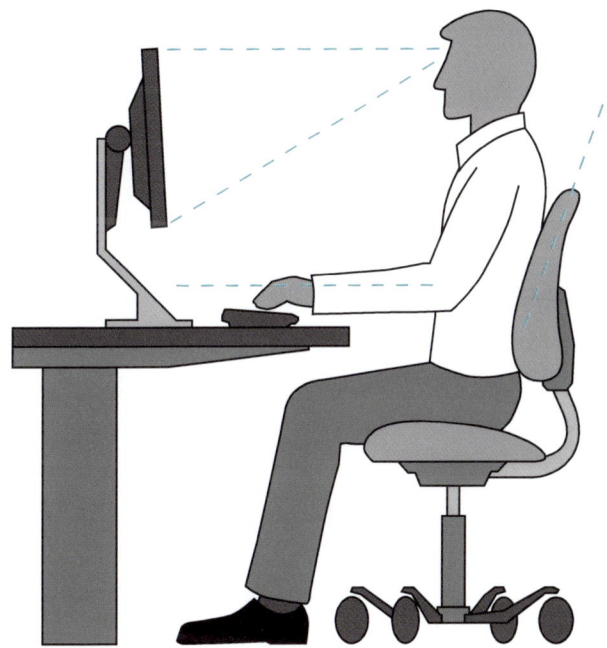

**Following are important considerations to set up and maintain neutral body postures while sitting at the computer workstation:**
- Your hands, wrists, and forearms are straight, in-line and roughly parallel to the floor.
- Your head is as vertical as possible, or bent only slightly forward.

THE BACK PAIN PERSONAL HEALTH PLAN 49

# PREVENTION AND TREATMENT

- Your shoulders are relaxed and upper arms hang naturally at the side of the body.
- Your elbows are close to the body.
- Your feet are supported by the floor or a footrest used to allow feet to be flat.
- Adjust the back rest of the chair so that it supports the curve in the low back.
- Adjust the height of the chair so that the level of the elbows is approximately the same height as the keyboard.
- Allow sufficient clearance to move knees and legs under the desk
- The thighs and hips are parallel to the floor, and supported by a well-padded seat.
- Your knees are approximately the same height as your hips with the feet slightly forward.
- Have the top of the screen at eye level.
- Reference material is easy to look at.

Regardless of how good your working posture is, working in the same position or sitting still for prolonged periods is not ideal. Small changes in your working position throughout the day can relieve stress, but care should be taken to maintain a neutral body position.

- You should break tasks up throughout the day to allow other muscles and joints to be used.
- Perform stretching exercises regularly throughout the day.
- Alternate between tasks that use different muscle groups.
- Also make sure that the other components of your work station support neutral body positioning including the mouse, keyboard, monitor and chair, and that they allow adjustability.
- Give your eyes a break by looking at a distant object regularly.

# PREVENTION AND TREATMENT

## When to seek medical advice

Although most back pain is resolved completely within a few weeks, it is important to know that it can still be caused by a more serious underlying disease.

So, if you experience any of the following, **please see your doctor immediately:**

- Pain caused by an injury or fall, which may indicate a fracture (especially if you have osteoporosis).
- Difficulty in controlling your bowels or bladder.
- Fever, chills, sweats or other signs that may be the result of an infection.
- Unexplained weight loss before or around the time of the back pain.
- Pain that is so intense you can't move around.
- Numbness in your leg, foot, groin, or rectal area, or a feeling like "pins and needles."
- Pain going down your leg to your thigh or below your knee.
- Pain that doesn't improve after two or three weeks.
- Pain that continues at night.
- If you have cancer or a strong family history of cancer; and/or if you are aged over sixty-five and have not experienced similar back pain before.

These symptoms could signal nerve damage or other serious medical problems and need to be investigated as soon as possible. The best advice is to have the cause assessed and get a correct diagnosis so that you can find the right treatment and pain relief.

If required your doctor may do further physical tests. However these tests are not recommended for non-specific back pain, especially if the pain is due to muscle or ligament strain.

# PREVENTION AND TREATMENT

## The three stages of lifestyle restoration

1. Learn the skills and methods to aid short-, medium-, and long-term recovery.
2. Take action! Modify and put into practise your newly learned skills.
3. Set goals. Your PHP is directly linked to motivate you to continue your action plan.

## The five skills of the back pain personal health plan

### SKILL 1: Mindset Skills

- Knowledge: the key to long lasting recovery.
- Recognising negative feelings and behaviours to your back pain.
- Understanding the cycle of chronic pain.
- Importance of a positive outlook and mindset.
- Altering pre-programmed pain patterns.
- Anatomy education.

### SKILL 2: Lifestyle Management Skills

- Pacing.
- Ergonomic advise.
- Daily activity changes.
- Avoiding muscle imbalance.
- Correct lifting techniques.
- Learning relaxation.
- Goal setting.
- Time management.

# PREVENTION AND TREATMENT

### SKILL 3: Pain Management Skills
- Team up with GP for pain medication review.
- Heat.
- Ice.
- TENS.
- Massage.
- Self massage techniques.
- Pacing.

### SKILL 4: Exercise Related Skills
- Condition specific/therapeutic exercise.
- Aerobic exercise programme.
- Postural strengthening.
- Learn how to stretch the spine.
- Learn how to strengthen the back.
- Education on importance of exercise.

### SKILL 5: Healthy Living Skills
- Quit smoking.
- Diet.
- Manage weight.

# EXERCISE GUIDE

"Nick Sinfield has put together a system for back rehabilitation that is easy to understand and easy to follow for the layman. The book highlights the essential aspects of neck and back health in a system that can be followed by even the most sedentary of individuals. I have found it a very useful tool in the rehabilitation and advancement of many people under my instruction."

*Trevor Chung*
*IFBB Certified Trainer, Mr Europe 2005 Bodybuilding Champion*

# EXERCISE GUIDE

The following exercises are compiled to supply you with the most effective stretches and strengthening exercises for your neck, back, legs and arms. Each exercise targets a specific area quickly to help you gain confidence and mobility quickly. The programme also includes graduated back strengthening exercises to achieve excellent core and spine stability.

This is a complete, self-managed exercise guide designed to improve your back pain through integrated mind and body rehabilitation. The aim of the exercise programme is to help you return to a full and physically active life with confidence. Building on the knowledge you gained in the first half of the programme the exercises will enable you to:

- Gain new understanding of how your spine and body works
- Increase your confidence in exercising
- Identify muscular tightness and imbalances
- Improve your posture
- Use stretching to ease the build-up of tense muscles
- Gradually strengthen your back muscles as you continue to gain confidence and regain your full range of activity

For many people, back pain is incredibly disabling, both in terms of the pain they experience and the restrictions the condition places on their mobility and independence. When someone has been in pain for months or even years, it often blots out their ability to think rationally about their condition. They feel panicked, fearful and pessimistic about the future of their health. It is at times like these that you need to keep in mind that pain does not equal harm.

# EXERCISE GUIDE

## The importance of pacing your return to exercise and fitness

If you have suffered from long term chronic back pain, you will need to start slowly when beginning the exercise programme, only performing a few repetitions and slowly increasing as you feel stronger. Think of it as a marathon, not a sprint. Slowly your confidence will improve and your muscles and joints will gain strength and mobility, allowing you to do the suggested number of repetitions. If you push your body too fast too soon, the ache in your muscles and joints will make you feel like giving up on the programme.

Just because you are in pain now, it doesn't mean that you are facing permanent disability or irreparable damage to your spine. As you discovered in the first part of this programme, to change how you feel, you may have to change how you act and behave in order to feel less back pain.

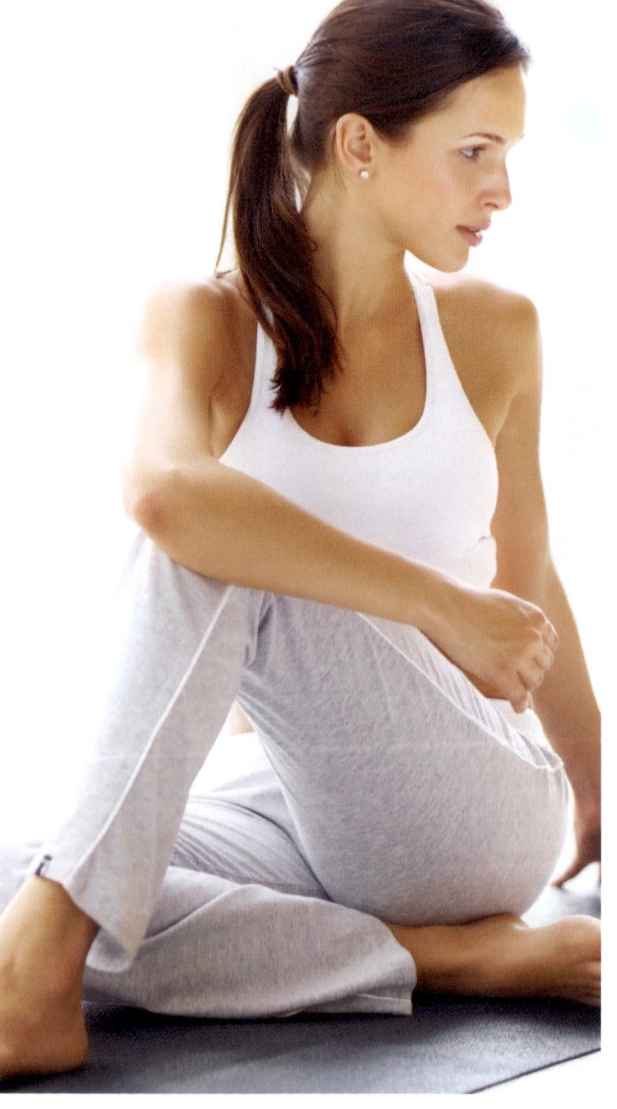

# EXERCISE GUIDE

The programme requires an open mind, discipline, concentration and total commitment to influence a real and lasting change in your back health. Because the programme is based on a mental realignment as well as physical strengthening, positive envisioning techniques and mental exercises play a major role.

Not everyone sees results immediately. Depending on the type of back problems you have and your ability to overcome your fears and address the emotional issues underlying your pain, it may take weeks or even months before you see a real improvement. However, you will see results if you follow the programme faithfully and commit to adjusting your mindset.

Let's begin!

# MENTAL REHABILITATION EXERCISES

One of the biggest hurdles back pain sufferers face in overcoming their affliction is developing confidence in the power of their own minds. Just as they fear the physical weakness of their spine and back muscles, they fear that their own minds are just not strong enough to overcome the pain. Your mind contains incredible power and you can harness that power to help your pain.

This is why a big part of the programme involves changing the way you think. By helping you build confidence in the power of your own mind, you will learn to see your back pain as a psychological, and physical issue. As such, it can be addressed by the power of the mind. By repeating key phrases that stimulate your mind to connect with the pain in positive ways, you will start the process of healing.

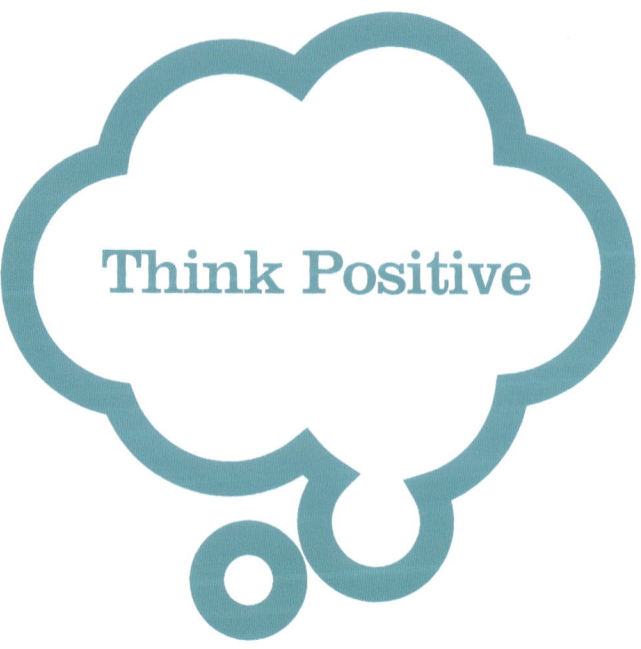

# MENTAL REHABILITAION EXERCISES

**Each day, say the following things to yourself (silently or aloud):**

- Structural abnormalities of the spine are the normal consequence of aging.
- My pain is a harmless condition which I will overcome.
- I can heal my pain through simple exercises, postural changes and renewed physical activity.
- I am not intimidated or afraid of my pain.
- By recognising and accepting self responsibility, I am well on my way to healing myself.
- I am in control of the pain, and I can choose to eliminate it by becoming more conscious of my pain patterns and negative behaviours.

With every day that passes, you will find it easier and easier to see the effect your mental reconditioning has on your ability to manage and reduce pain.

If you find that you experience a setback, or just want a little extra support, it helps to discuss your programme with a healthcare professional

# BREATHING EXERCISE

**Aim:** To develop deeper, more relaxed, healthier breathing patterns

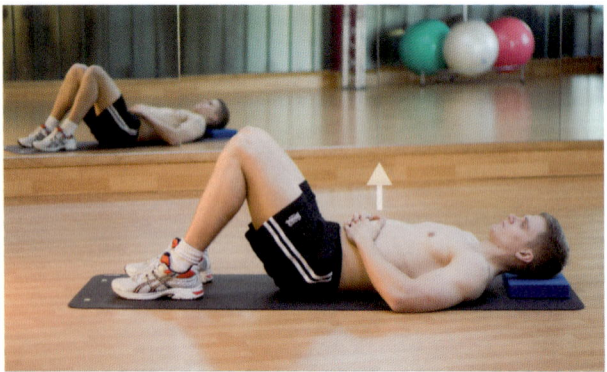
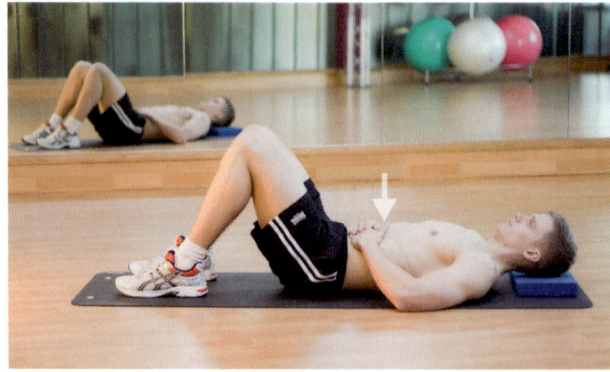

## Starting Position:

Lie on your back on a mat or the carpet. Place a small, flat cushion or book under your head. Bend your knees and keep your feet straight and in line with your hips. Place your hands on your stomach. Keep your chest and ribcage relaxed and your chin gently tucked in.

## Action:

1. Breathe in through the nose.
2. Feel your stomach filling with air and rising up.
3. Keep your head, neck and shoulders relaxed.
4. Ensure your shoulders are not rising as you breathe.
5. Breathe out through the mouth and feel your stomach flatten.

Repeat this breathing exercise throughout the day, in the car, office or at home, whenever you feel tension building.

### Watch points
- Do not tense up through the neck and shoulders.
- Concentrate on using your diaphragm to breath.
- Imagine a small weight on your breastbone keeping it relaxed during the exercise.

# MUSCLE IMBALANCE

A basic understanding of how our bodies work should be common knowledge for all of us, but it isn't!

If we have a nagging ache or pain, we should know how to stretch that area or muscle in order to aid the healing process. Unfortunately, most of us don't know how to use stretching exercises to address the onset of pain and keep ourselves limber.

Instead, most of us become less flexible as we get older. We start noticing that we can't touch our toes anymore, and one day we realise we even have difficulty putting socks on! Our muscles seem to tighten and tense up like boards.

You may be surprised to hear that age isn't the main culprit. A muscle's natural reaction is to contract. Muscles contract as a defense mechanism when they sense the onset of pain. In this way, our bodies develop habitual patterns of pain, which can also trigger a spasm attack.

Your muscles need balanced strength and flexibility to support your body height and weight and allow for normal movement. Unfortunately, for most of us, keeping all the muscles equally balanced is a tall order. We work some of our muscles too hard and allow other muscles to weaken, creating strength imbalances. We also over-stretch some of our muscles whilst leaving others to contract and become tense and tight. All of these tendencies lead to imbalanced posture over time.

Unfortunately, most people have no idea they're using their bodies in a way that creates imbalance. Let's look at some of the most common reasons for physical imbalance:

# MUSCLE IMBALANCE

### Lack of stretching

Most of us who do certain activities for long periods over and over again will lose flexibility if we don't adopt a regular stretching routine. This is because doing activities for extended periods of time cause some muscles to stay in a short, contracted state permanently, whilst others overstretch to compensate and become vulnerable to tearing and damage. Suddenly, we can no longer touch our toes or, in extreme cases, even our knees! To start your recovery, you need to address the muscle imbalances that causes conditions such as muscular tightness, disc herniation or spondylosis in the first place.

### Sedentary lifestyle

If you sit for long periods, your muscles, tendons, and ligaments will adapt to this position. The result of this shortening causes tightness around joints, nerves or lengthened muscles that overstrain, creating imbalances in the body.

If you regularly spend long periods of time in front of a computer or television, behind the wheel, or at a desk writing or reading, the result will most likely be the weakening and stretching of your back muscles, rounded shoulders and a neck position that tilts or cranes forward. These effects lead to poor postures and muscle imbalances.

If you must lead a sedentary lifestyle, you need to sit with a square, straight-on posture, elbows by your sides, neck long and shoulder blades drawn into your spine. Make sure you get up at least once an hour to walk around, stretch, and loosen up. Get a glass of water, take a walk outside, perform a handful of stretches, or visit a colleague — anything to get your body moving.

# MUSCLE IMBALANCE

## Left- or right-handedness

Because so many of us are either left or right-handed, we tend to use one side of our bodies more than the other during our daily activities. This strengthens some muscles and leaves others underdeveloped and weak. To create a better balance throughout the body and better support for the spine and the back, start consciously using both sides of your body more evenly.

If you normally lift your child with your right arm, for example, or balance her on your right hip, try lifting her with your left arm and balancing her on your left hip. Bend your knees when lifting her and never carry her for too long on just one side. Get used to shifting and using more of your muscles. This will improve your overall body symmetry, strength and flexibility.

Most of us also tend to carry our possessions on one side, which can also cause problems. For instance, habitually wearing a shoulder bag on one shoulder causes your body to tilt and bend to compensate, straining your spine. It also forces the muscles on the carrying side to work harder than the ones on the other side. If you need to carry some sort of bag on your shoulder, be sure to frequently switch sides, so both shoulders are worked equally. Even better: use a rucksack that allows you to achieve balance between both sides of your body.

These chronic muscle imbalances are a major contributing factor to back pain. However, with the help of the exercises later in the book, you can self-assess the strength and flexibility of your muscle pairs in your hips, pelvis, spine, and throughout the body. The idea is to find out which muscles are strong and which are weak, which are tight and which are more flexible, and which may

## MUSCLE IMBALANCE

be overworked or shortened. Since these various imbalances stress joints, other muscles, and ligaments, the goal of the therapy is to rebalance the muscles so that each muscle pair is as close to "normal" as possible. By evening out the muscle tension between the left and right sides of the body or between the front and back, the body supports the spine more evenly, automatically improving posture. This postural realignment allows the vertebrae to move back into position, taking pressure off irritated nerves and muscles and eliminating back pain.

As you can now see, your back pain is caused by a multitude of factors brought on over many years by physical and mental habits which have become the norm for your body. It will take time to break the cycle, but it can be done. Once you establish new, healthier daily physical and mental habits, you will start to feel in control of your pain.

# POSTURAL AWARENESS

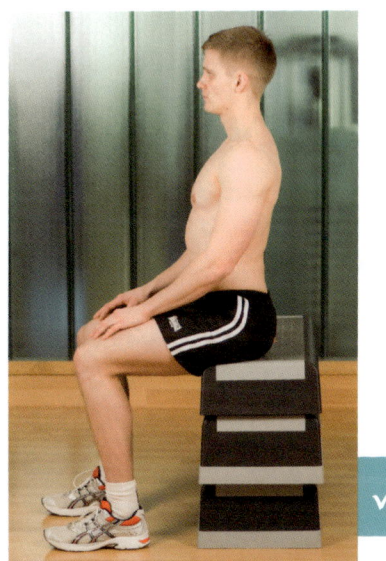

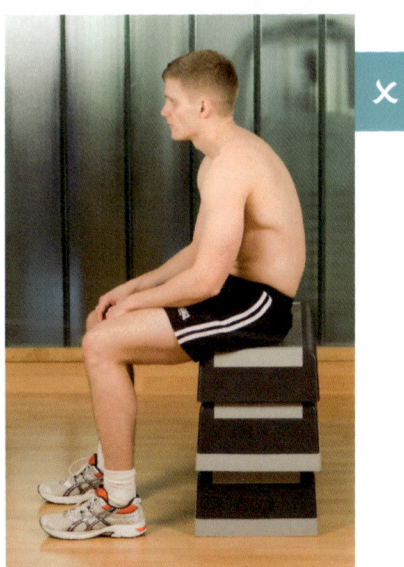

## Postural awareness

Developing a keen awareness of your posture is one of the most effective ways you can strengthen your back and reduce muscle tension. Of course, the majority of us do not have perfect posture, and the misalignment of our spines can create imbalances resulting in pain. When standing or sitting, it's important to be aware of any imbalances in the muscles or areas of stress. Once you develop this awareness, you can address these issues by adjusting your posture and practising the exercises to reinforce better posture. As your sitting and standing habits improve, you'll notice far less tension in your body and less strain on you soft tissues and spine.

**Slumping:** If you tend to slump in your chair, it generally means your low back is overstretched. As a result, your muscles and joints compensate, causing shortening to the soft tissues and imbalances throughout the spine.

THE BACK PAIN PERSONAL HEALTH PLAN    65

# POSTURAL AWARENESS

Let's look at this cycle in more depth.

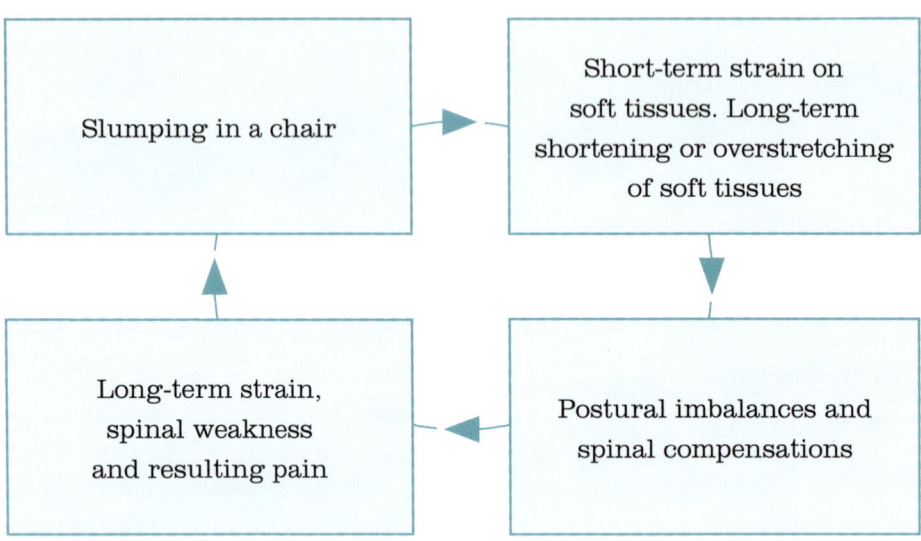

## Prolonged sitting postures

When we remain seated for long periods of time (for instance, seated at the computer or driving long distances), it can cause our muscles to contract and tighten, resulting in pain. Regular changes of position and gentle stretching, ideally every hour, will benefit our muscles and joints.

## Uneven sitting postures

If you sit consistently with your legs crossed to a particular side, it can cause your lower back to curve sideways, putting strain on your soft tissues. Try switching sides each time you cross your legs to create more balance in your sitting posture.

# POSTURAL AWARENESS

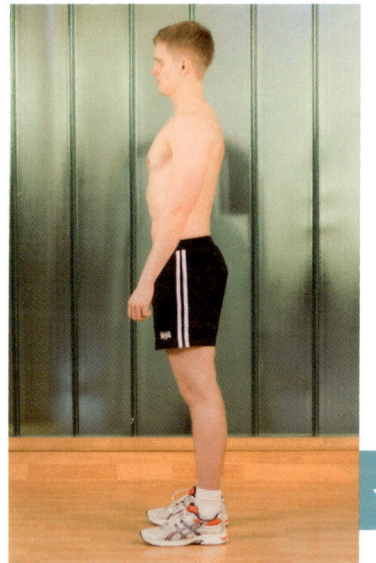

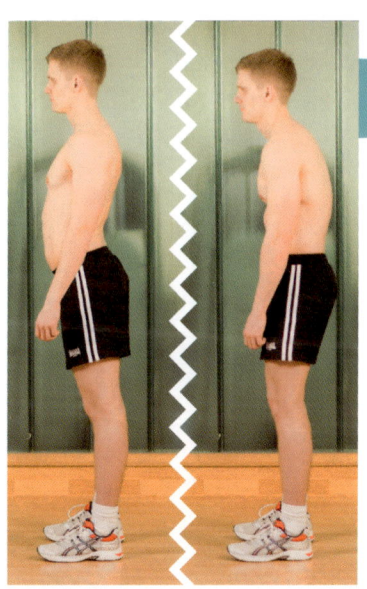

## Standing posture

To determine whether your standing posture needs to be adjusted, stand in front of a full-length mirror. Stand sideways, and place your hands on your hip bones. Now, imagine your pelvis were a bowl of water, and feel the position of your hip bones. Are you tipping the "bowl" forwards or backwards, or are you holding it level? For ideal posture, you want to focus on keeping the imaginary bowl of water level. Focus on making slight postural adjustments until you achieve this effect. Now take a mental snapshot of how this looks, and remember how it feels to hold the posture.

Next, look at the way you hold your head and neck. You want to make sure your chin is tucked in slightly towards your chest, so that your neck is lengthened slightly. If your chin or head juts forward, gently pull yourself into alignment.

And finally, develop an awareness of whether you tend to favour one leg or another when you stand. If there is an imbalance in the way you distribute weight on your legs, make sure you change your weight-bearing leg regularly.

THE BACK PAIN PERSONAL HEALTH PLAN    67

# POSTURAL STRENGTHENING

## Postural strengthening

Now that you have a greater awareness of your postural issues, you can begin to address those issues by strengthening your areas of weakness. Improving your posture through strengthening exercises is key to eliminating soft tissue imbalance and resulting pain. As part of your rehabilitation programme, commit to achieving these postural corrections throughout the day. If you can find healthier ways to stand and sit, it can radically change your back pain. After all, most people spend more hours in the day standing and sitting than they do in more active pursuits. Improving these two postural modes form an essential part of your overall back health.

"Protruding" posture exercises: If your abdomen and buttocks tend to protrude when you stand, it increases the arch in your lower back, creating imbalances in the muscles. To improve your posture, practice the Pelvic tilts exercise on page 85 which can be done anywhere, at any time: using your abdominal muscles, gently tilt your pelvis backward and tuck in your tailbone. Repeat as many times as you like. This simple exercise helps realign a protruding posture and allows the back to relax.

Other helpful exercises for a protruding posture include:

- Knee to chest stretch ..... 75
- Bottom to heels stretch ..... 77
- Kneeling quad stretch ..... 98
- Bridging Level 1 ..... 90
- Chin tucks, shoulder blade and neck strengthening ..... 109 - 110
- Low back strengthening exercises ..... 83 - 96

# POSTURAL STRENGTHENING

"Slumped" posture exercises: If you tend to slump forward when you stand, with your pelvis tilted backwards and your tailbone tucked under, you have a "slumped' posture. This posture can cause your shoulders to collapse inward, creating tension and pain. To improve your posture, try imagining that there is a string attached to the crown of your head, and that the string is being pulled upwards tautly. Allow the string to slowly pull you taller and straighter. Tuck in your chin, draw your shoulder blades down into your back, lift your chest and allow your neck to lengthen.

Other helpful exercises for a slumped posture include:

- Back extensions — 80
- Bridging Level 1 — 90
- Chin tucks, shoulder blade and neck strengthening — 109 - 110
- Low back strengthening exercises Level 1 — 83 - 91
- Hamstring and calf stretches — 99, 101

# BACK PAIN TREATMENTS

This selection of treatments can help you manage pain whilst you focus on strengthening mental control over your pain and your exercise programme. Although the ultimate aim of the programme is to help you become pain-free so that you don't need these pain-management treatments, they are helpful to use as short-term, interim pain relief.

Cold treatment: Using ice packs on painful areas helps to reduce inflammation and calm the pain receptors. Apply ice for 10 minutes and repeat every two hours as needed.

*(Precautions: wrap ice in thin towelling; if icing irritates symptoms, discontinue the treatment; if you have heart, circulatory or lung problems, decreased sensation or an open wound, consult a healthcare professional before commencing ice pack treatment.)*

Heat treatment: Use heat packs, such as wheat bags, to help relax muscle spasms and tension. Apply heat pack for 20 minutes and repeat every two hours as needed. Even a hot shower over the painful area can help ease muscle tension.

*(Precautions: use protective layers to protect the skin from excessive heat; follow the instructions on the heating product; if you have heart, circulatory or lung problems, decreased sensation or an open wound, consult a healthcare professional before commencing heat treatment.)*

Soft tissue massage or self-massage: Gentle massage from a qualified massage therapist can help with pain relief. Self-massage can also be helpful. Try standing against the wall or lying on the floor and massage your muscles using tennis balls pressed gently between your tissues and the hard surface. A vibrating, hand-held massage device can also help relieve muscle tension and pain.

Bending and lifting advice: To use the right postural technique when bending and lifting, keep your feet shoulder width apart, bend your knees, and keep your chest up and your back straight. If you are lifting a heavy or awkward object, bend the knees and go into a half-kneeling position, keeping the weight drawn close to your chest. Never lift heavy objects repeatedly over a short period of time.

# EXERCISE GUIDE

As you begin performing the exercises, aim to connect to your body mentally. When you stretch a muscle, concentrate on the sensation this creates within that muscle. Only move and stretch as far as is comfortable, and only take yourself into a position where you can breathe and relax into the movement.

Always listen to your body and learn the difference between the feeling you get when you stretch a tight sore muscle and the pain caused when you hurt yourself. If you feel a sharp stabbing pain when exercising, stop immediately.

These exercises will teach you discipline and control, and help you to connect your mind to your muscles. Ultimately, this will lead to you achieving the result that you want...less pain!

This exercise programme will take you from doing no back exercises to doing 20-30 minutes a day, enough to increase the flexibility and strength of your back and neck.

You may need to gradually increase the repetitions until you are able to follow the recommended amount. But if you persevere, you will gradually improve.
Everyone is different, so adjust the exercises to fit your needs. If your neck and shoulder blades are the main problem, then concentrate on this area on a daily basis.

To help achieve the correct technique, each exercise is accompanied with a Watch Points section. To perform these exercises safely, make sure you check this section for each exercise.

The General Aerobic Exercise Programme will give you the confidence to get moving again and the motivation to return to those neglected pastimes you have been missing.

The most important consideration when learning these exercises is safety. If you have any health problems or concerns, you must consult a health care professional before you start the programme.

# EXCERCISE PROGRAMME

> **"** I would recommend this book to anyone suffering with long-term back and neck pain, it includes great educational content and easy to follow exercises. **"**

*Stuart Wain, Managing Director US Investment Bank*

# TOP TIPS

- Follow the instructions for each exercise closely. You must learn the proper technique to achieve the best results.

- Keep an open mind. As you learn each exercise, your body will surprise you. Some stretches will feel difficult, some easy and some tight only on one side of your body! Adjust and adapt as you progress through the programme.

- Keep challenging your body. If you feel able to increase the repetitions, sets or levels for each exercise, then go for it.

- You must exercise consistently. Build a daily routine and stick with the programme. No excuses!

- Mix it up! Vary the exercises considerably during each week. Focus sometimes on stretches, sometimes on strength, sometimes general fitness. This will help keep you interested and motivated.

- Remember to work on your mental resilience at the same time as your physical programme. You must believe that your pain will get better.

- To keep yourself motivated, reward yourself with a little present if you complete the exercises each day for a month.

- When exercising, focus on the movements. Do not allow yourself to become distracted by anything or anyone.

- Be patient. We all get frustrated at not progressing faster at one time or another. Give your body the chance over the long term to reach your goals.

- Be realistic. You may not achieve a 100% pain free life. But you will achieve substantially less pain during your daily activities if you stick to your exercise programme.

# LOW BACK STRETCHES

The stretches in this section focus on your low back. Over time, they help you improve the range of motion in your back in order to make everyday tasks easier.

## Benefits of low back stretching
- ✓ Reduced tension in your muscles and joints
- ✓ Improved posture
- ✓ Less discomfort in your lower back
- ✓ A more comfortable body to walk around in all day

## The Routine

- If you suffer from low back pain, start off by practising each exercise to uncover any muscular tightness to the spine.
- Identify three to five exercises that you feel best stretch your problem areas.
- Do this routine every day.
- Follow each exercise instruction and gradually increase to the recommended amount.
- Keep each motion slow and controlled.
- Remember to maintain abdominal breathing throughout the exercises.

LOW BACK STRETCHES

# KNEE TO CHEST STRETCH

**Aim:** To improve flexibility of your low back

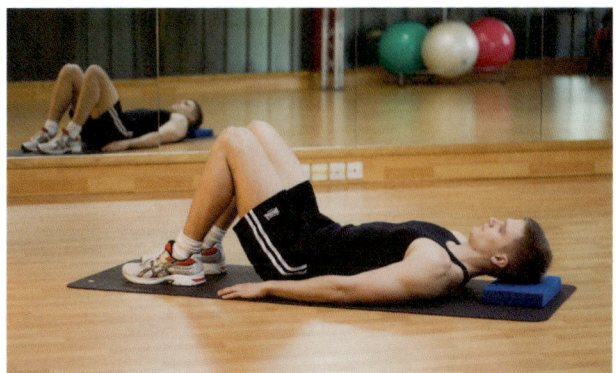 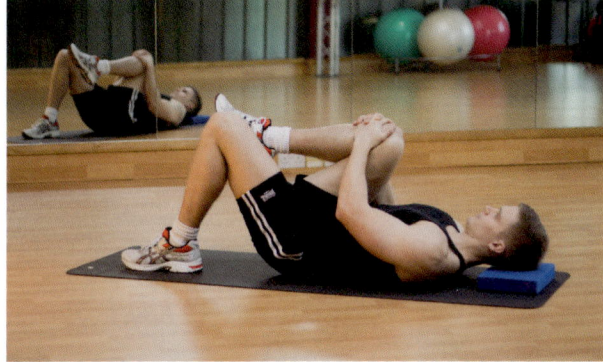

### Starting Position:

Lie on your back on a mat or the carpet. Place a small flat cushion or book under your head. Bend your knees and keep your feet straight and in line with your hips. Keep your chest and ribcage relaxed and your chin gently tucked in.

### Action:

Bend one knee up towards your chest and grasp with two hands behind your knee. Slowly increase this stretch as comfort allows. Hold for 20-30 seconds with controlled deep breaths.

**Repeat three times, alternating legs.**

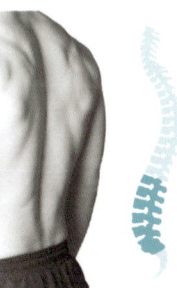

**Watch points**
- Do not tense up through the neck, chest or shoulders
- Only stretch as far as is comfortable

**Variations:** Grasp behind both knees and stretch into chest

THE BACK PAIN PERSONAL HEALTH PLAN

LOW BACK STRETCHES

# CAT STRETCH

**Aim:** To mobilise and stretch the entire spine

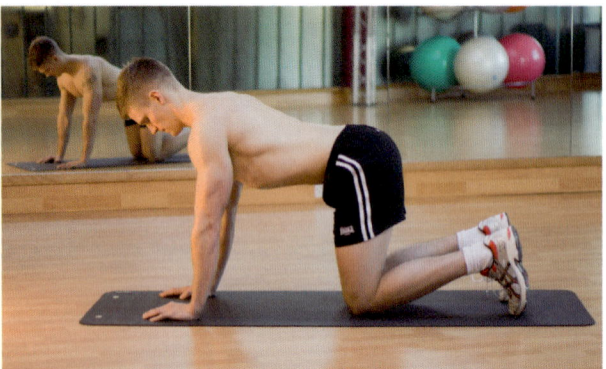 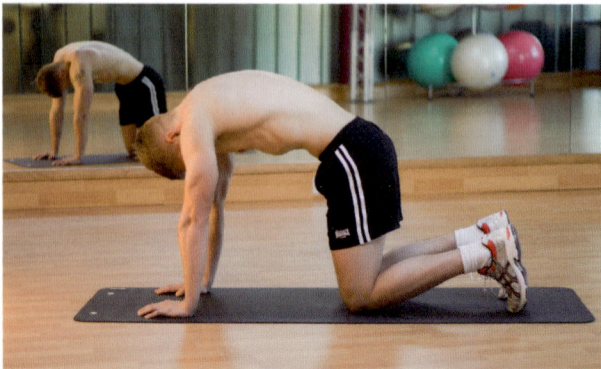

## Starting Position:

Kneel on all fours, with your knees under hips and hands under shoulders. Make sure you keep a small inward curve in your low back. Keep your neck long, your shoulder blades down and your elbows unlocked.

## Action:

Begin at the base of your spine, slowly tuck your tailbone under, work your way up the spine finishing with your chin on your chest and your spine in a C-shaped curve. Slowly uncurl the spine, leading from the tailbone vertebra by vertebra until you return to the starting position.

**Repeat eight to 10 times.**

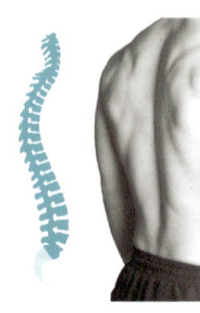

### Watch points
- Concentrate on moving every vertebra segment by segment.
- Do not overarch downwards or lift up your head.

LOW BACK STRETCHES

# BOTTOM TO HEELS STRETCH

**Aim:** To stretch and mobilise the spine

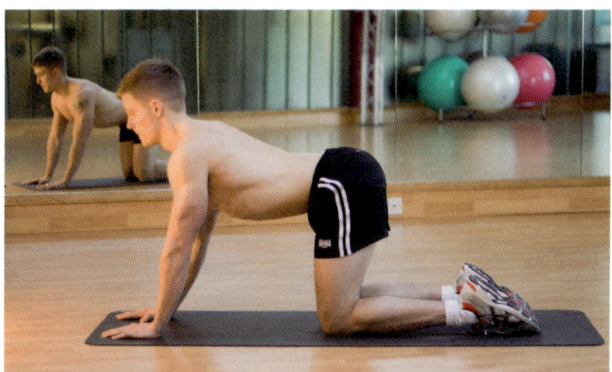 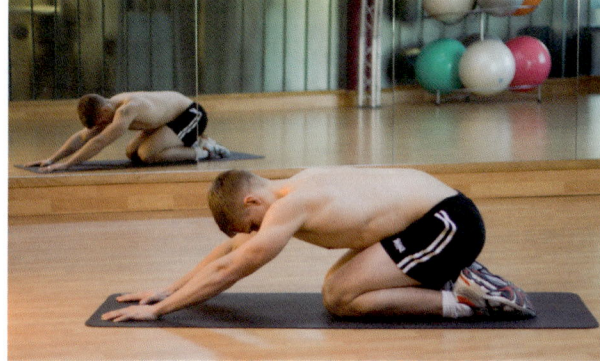

### Starting Position:

Kneel on all fours, with your knees under hips and hands under shoulders. Make sure you keep a small inward curve in your low back. Keep your neck long, your shoulder blades down and your elbows unlocked.

### Action:

Slowly take your bottom backwards keeping the natural curves in the spine. Only stretch as far as is comfortable. Hold the stretch for one deep breath and return to the starting position

**Repeat eight to 10 times.**

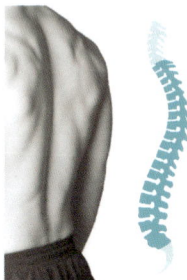

**Watch points**
- Avoid sitting back on your heels if you have a knee problem.
- Check your spinal alignment during the exercise with the help of a mirror.

THE BACK PAIN PERSONAL HEALTH PLAN    77

LOW BACK STRETCHES

# KNEE ROLLS

Aim: To stretch and mobilise the spine

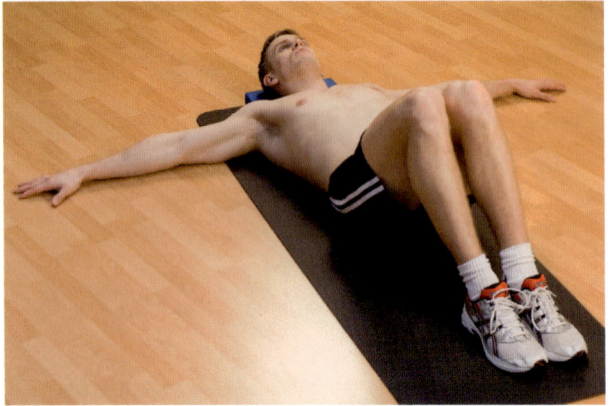

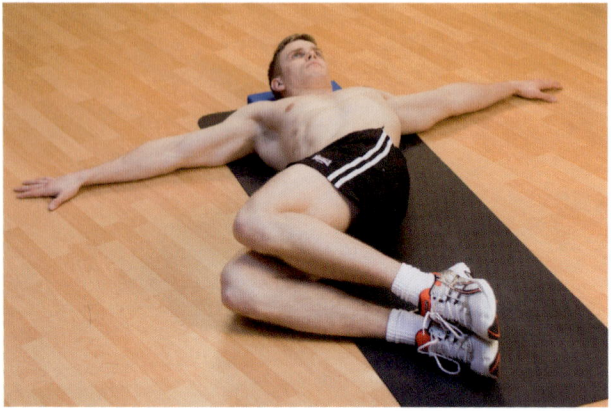

## Starting Position:

Lie on your back on a mat or the carpet. Place a small flat cushion or book under your head. Keep your knees bent and together. Keep your chest and ribcage relaxed and your chin gently tucked in.

## Action:

Roll your knees to one side, followed by your pelvis, keeping both shoulders on the floor. Hold the stretch for one deep breath and return to the starting position.

Repeat eight to 10 times, alternating sides.

### Watch points
- Do not move into pain only move as far as is comfortable.
- Place a pillow between your knees for comfort.

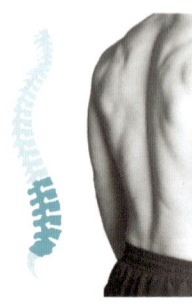

LOW BACK STRETCHES

# SCIATIC MOBILISING STRETCH

**Aim:** To mobilise the sciatic nerve and hamstrings

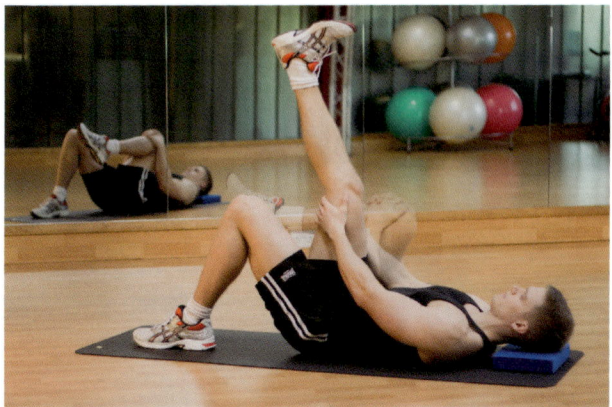

## Starting Position:

Lie on your back on a mat or the carpet. Place a small flat cushion or book under your head. Bend your knees and keep your feet straight and in line with your hips. Keep your chest and ribcage relaxed and your chin gently tucked in.

## Action:

Bend one knee upwards towards your chest and grasp with both hands behind the knee. Slowly straighten the knee whilst bringing your foot towards you. Hold for 20-30 seconds taking deep breathes. Bend the knee and return to the starting position.

**Repeat alternating legs two or three times.**

### Warning!

If you suffer from **sciatica**, please seek advice from a medical professional before attempting this exercise.

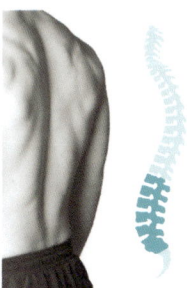

### Watch points
- Do not press your low back down into the floor as you stretch.
- Only stretch as far as is comfortable, and stop immediately if you feel pain, numbness or tingling

THE BACK PAIN PERSONAL HEALTH PLAN

LOW BACK STRETCHES

# BACK EXTENSIONS

Aim: To stretch and mobilise the spine backwards into extension

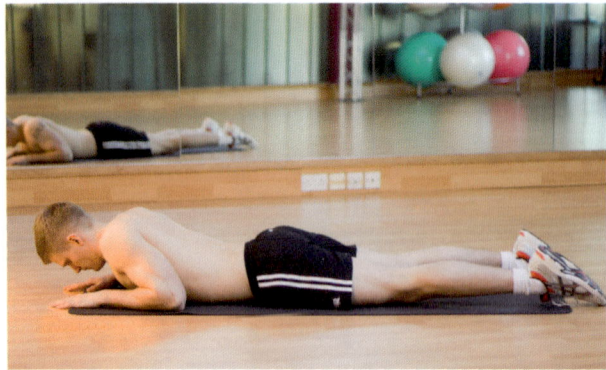 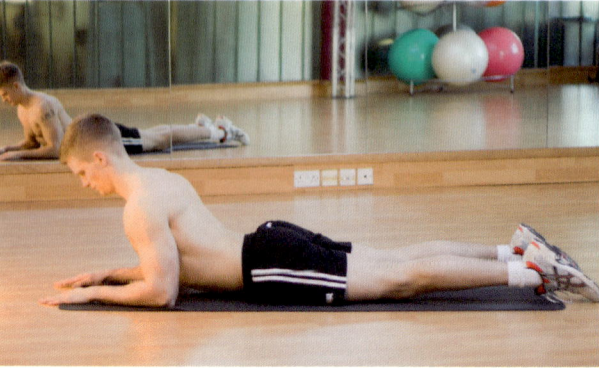

## Starting Position:

Lie on your stomach, and prop yourself on your elbows extending your spine. Keep your neck long.

## Action:

Gently keeping your neck long, extend your spine backwards, straightening your elbows if this feels comfortable. Hold for five to 10 seconds. Return to the starting position.

**Repeat eight to 10 times.**

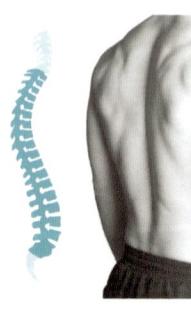

**Watch points**
- Do not extend your neck backwards.
- Only extend as far as is comfortable.

LOW BACK STRETCHES

# STANDING SIDE BENDS

**Aim:** To stretch the sides of the spine

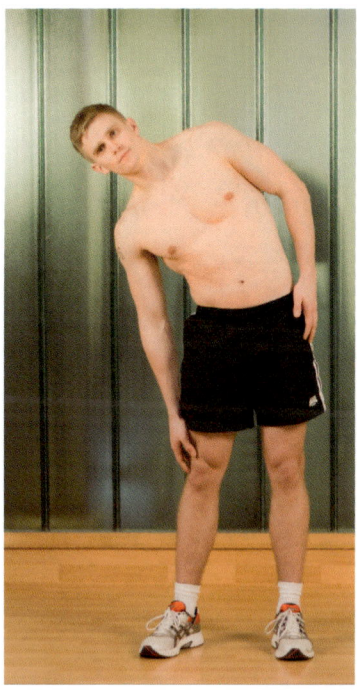
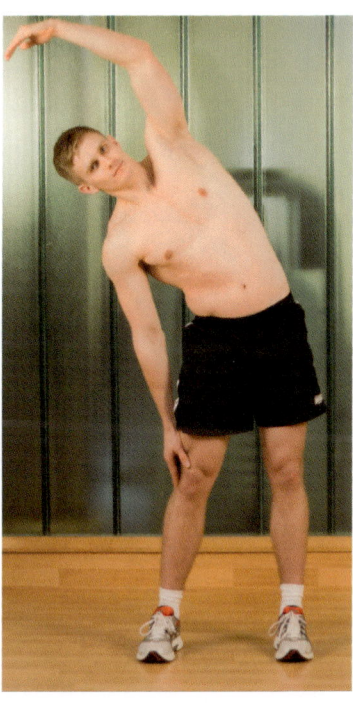

## Starting Position:

Stand with your feet hip-distance apart and your spine in alignment. Place one hand on your hip and the other on the outside of the thigh. Keep equal weight through both feet during the exercise. Keep your neck long.

## Action:

Slide the hand down the outside of the thigh, feeling the stretch on the opposite side. Return to the starting position.

**Repeat, alternating sides eight to 10 times.**

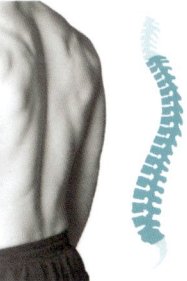

### Watch points
- Only stretch as far as is comfortable.
- Take deep abdominal breaths throughout the exercise.
- Keep your weight equally distributed through both feet throughout
- Keep upright and do not bend forwards

**Variations:** Instead of keeping one hand on your hip, raise the arm above the head to increase the stretch.

THE BACK PAIN PERSONAL HEALTH PLAN    81

LOW BACK STRETCHES

# SPINE ROTATIONS

Aim: To rotate the spine

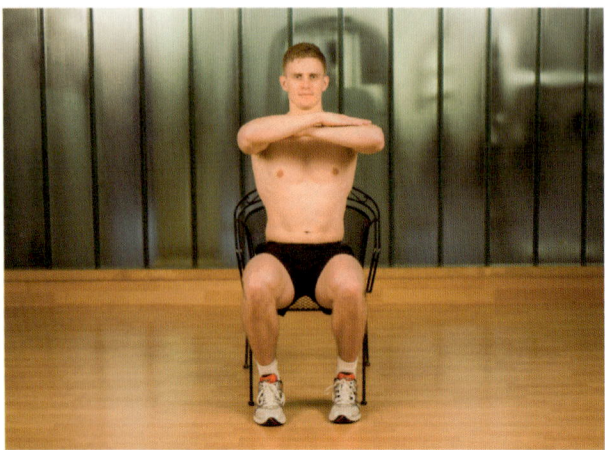 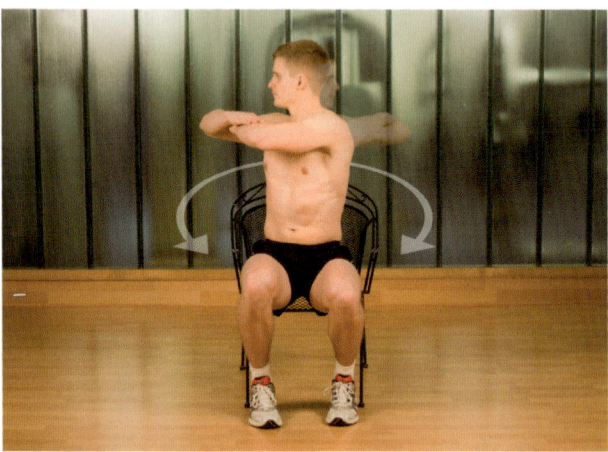

### Starting Position:

Sit in a chair and fold your arms in front of you, in line with your chest. Keep your shoulders down and your neck long. Imagine a metal pole down your spine, which you rotate around.

### Action:

Rotate to one side as far as is comfortable, whilst keeping your pelvis square. Slowly return to the starting position.

**Repeat 8-10 times alternating sides**

### Watch points
- Keep equal weight through both buttocks.
- Concentrate on pivoting around the imaginary pole.
- Keep your shoulders down and neck long

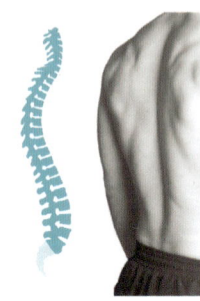

# LOW BACK STRENGTHENING

**LEVEL 1**

In Level 1 of your strengthening programme, you will learn how to activate your deep abdominal muscles, low back muscles and buttocks. This will give you a solid foundation of muscles around your back in order to avoid further injury or re-occurrence.

## Benefits of low back stretching
- ✓ Less discomfort in your lower back
- ✓ Everyday tasks will become easier
- ✓ More confidence in your back to take on new challenges
- ✓ Improved posture

## The Routine

- Start the Level 1 exercises and follow each exercise instruction and gradually increase to the recommended amount.
- Keep each motion slow and controlled.
- Remember to retain the abdominal breathing throughout the exercises.
- Between exercises, try to rest for no longer than five seconds.
- Even if you find Level 1 easy, make a point of practising these exercises every day for at least two weeks. It is important to lay a firm groundwork before progressing to Level 2.
- If you need more time, stick with Level 1 beyond the first two weeks.
- After two weeks, if you have achieved the recommended repetitions and sets, you can progress confidently to Level 2.

### LEVEL 1 — LOW BACK STRENGTHENING

# DEEP ABDOMINAL STRENGTHENING

**Aim:** To strengthen the deep supporting muscles surrounding the spine

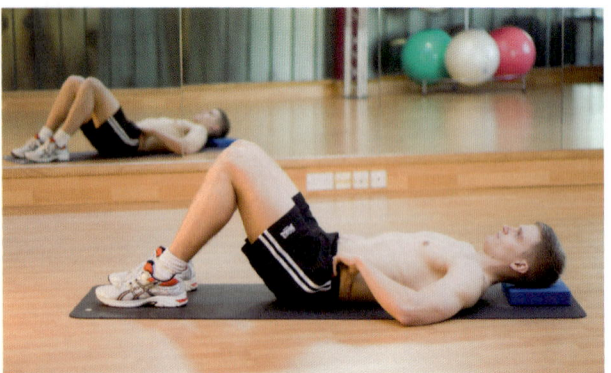 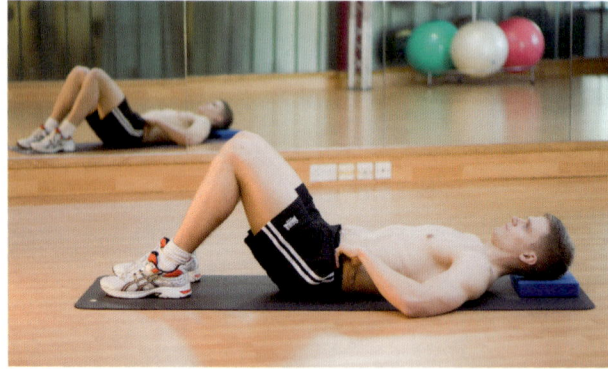

## Starting Position:

Lie on your back on a mat or the carpet. Place a small, flat cushion or book under your head. Bend your knees and keep your feet straight and in line with your hips. Keep your chest and ribcage relaxed and your chin gently tucked in. Once you have mastered this technique, keep practising in differing positions throughout the day.

## Action:

As you breathe out, draw up the muscles of the pelvic floor and lower abdominals, as though you were doing up an imaginary internal zipper! Hold this gentle muscle contraction whilst practising your abdominal breathing for five to 10 breaths.

**Repeat five times**

### Watch points
- Remember, this is a slow, gentle tightening of the deep abdominal muscles. Do not pull these muscles in using more than 25 per cent of your maximum strength.
- Make sure you do not tense up through the neck, shoulders or legs.

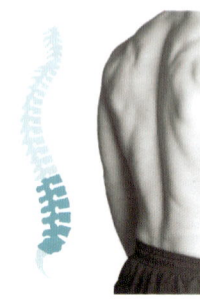

*LOW BACK STRENGTHENING*   **LEVEL 1**

# PELVIC TILTS

**Aim:** To stretch and strengthen the low back

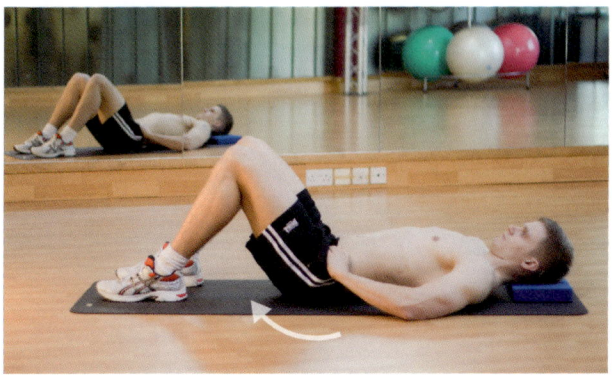 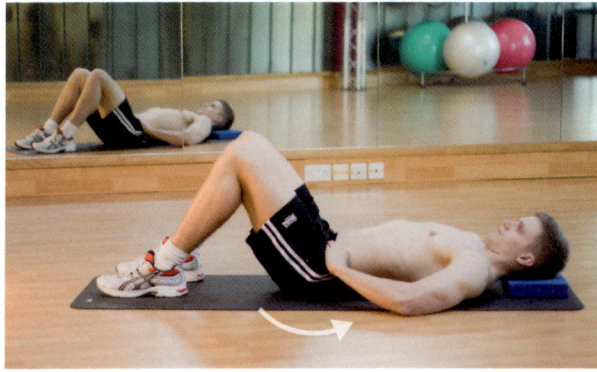

## Starting Position:

Lie on your back on a mat or the carpet. Place a small, flat cushion or book under your head. Bend your knees and keep your feet straight and in line with your hips. Keep your chest and ribcage relaxed and your chin gently tucked in.

## Action:

Gently tuck your tailbone under you whilst simultaneously contracting your stomach muscles. Feel your ribcage draw towards your pelvis and your low back gently press down into the mat. Now, return to the starting position and then slowly arch your back, feeling the low back muscles working.

**Repeat eight to 10 times**

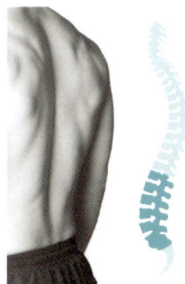

**Watch points**
- Only stretch as far as is comfortable.
- Take deep abdominal breaths throughout the exercise.
- Do not push down through you feet during the exercise.

**Modifications:** Place one hand on your stomach and the other under your low back and use this feedback to feel the correct muscles working.

# LEVEL 1 — LOW BACK STRENGTHENING
## LEG SLIDES

**Aim:** To strengthen the supporting muscles surrounding the spine

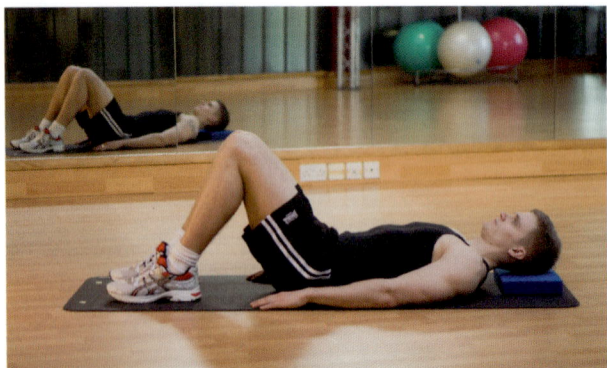
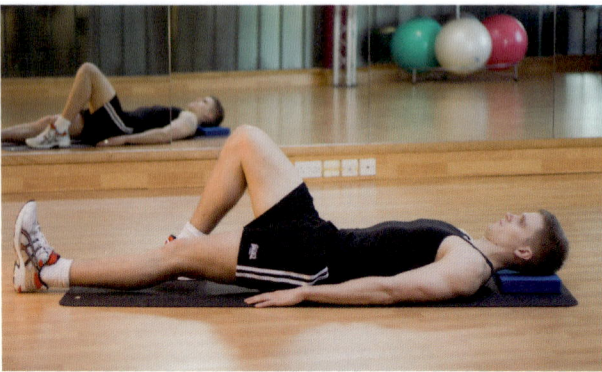

### Starting Position:

Lie on your back on a mat or the carpet. Place a small, flat cushion or book under your head. Bend your knees and keep your feet straight and in line with your hips. Keep your chest and ribcage relaxed and your chin gently tucked in.

### Action:

Slide one leg along the floor, keeping your back still and deep abdominals engaged. Return the leg to the bent position whilst carefully keeping your low back still.

**Repeat eight to 10 times, alternating legs.**

### Watch points
- Keep your deep abdominals activated throughout
- Do not let your low back arch
- Do not tense up through the chest, shoulders or neck

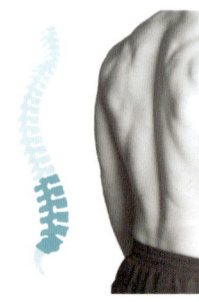

LOW BACK STRENGTHENING  LEVEL 1

# KNEE DROPS

**Aim:** To strengthen the supporting muscles surrounding the spine

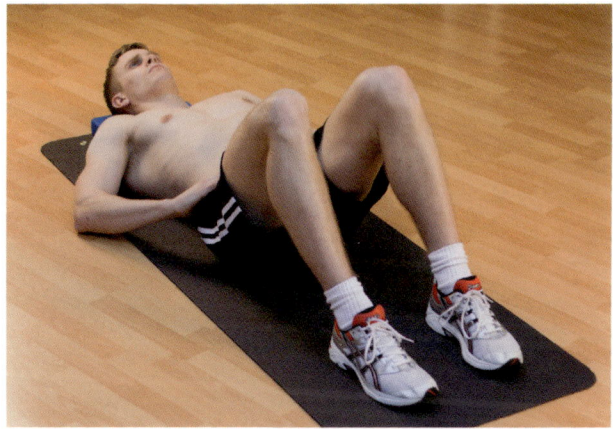
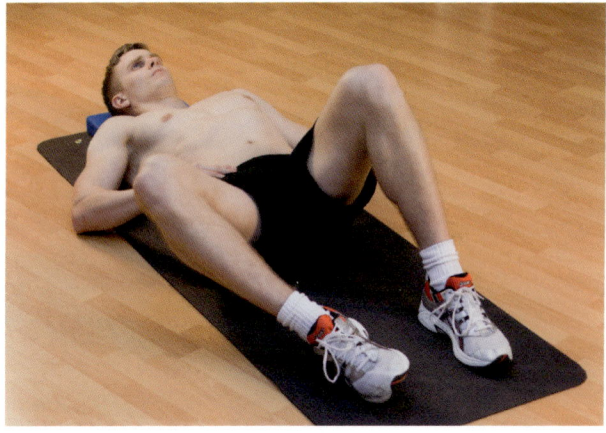

## Starting Position:

Lie on your back on a mat or the carpet. Place a small, flat cushion or book under your head. Bend your knees and keep your feet straight and in line with your hips. Keep your chest and ribcage relaxed and your chin gently tucked in.

## Action:

Allow one knee to drop slowly outwards whilst keeping your pelvis stationary. Draw the knee back in towards your body.

**Repeat eight to 10 times, alternating legs.**

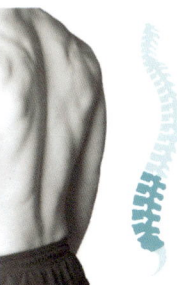

### Watch points
- Keep your deep abdominals activated throughout
- Imagine a spirit level across your hipbones and keep this level at all times
- Do not tense up through the chest, shoulders or neck

THE BACK PAIN PERSONAL HEALTH PLAN

### LEVEL 1 — LOW BACK STRENGTHENING
# LEG LIFTS

**Aim:** To strengthen the supporting muscles surrounding the spine

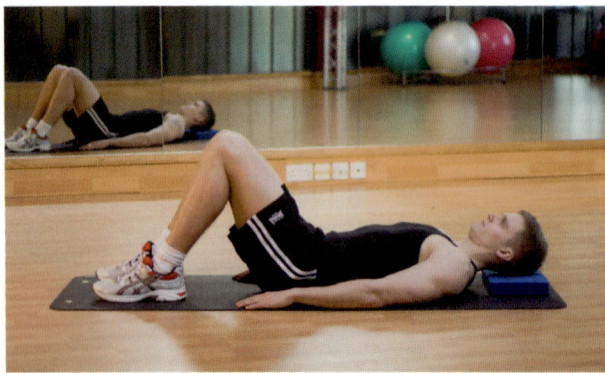 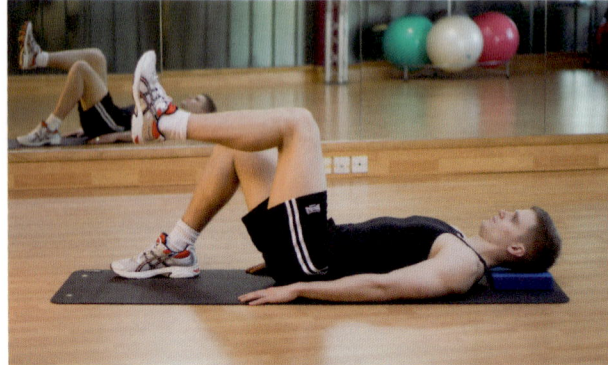

## Starting Position:

Lie on your back on a mat or the carpet. Place a small, flat cushion or book under your head. Bend your knees and keep your feet straight and in line with your hips. Keep your chest and ribcage relaxed and your chin gently tucked in.

## Action:

Slide one foot back and then lift this leg up until your lower leg is horizontal. Lower the leg to the starting position.

**Repeat eight to 10 times, alternating legs.**

### Watch points
- Keep your deep abdominals activated throughout.
- Do not let your low back arch.
- Do not tense up through the chest, shoulders or neck.
- Make sure you do not tense up through the neck, shoulders or legs.

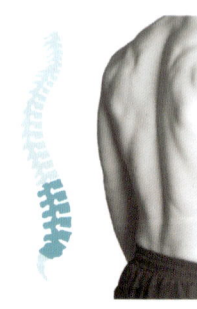

LOW BACK STRENGTHENING · LEVEL 1

# SWIMMING

**Aim:** To strengthen the low back and buttocks

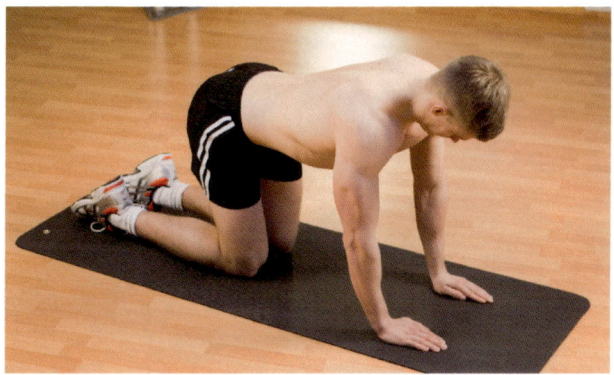 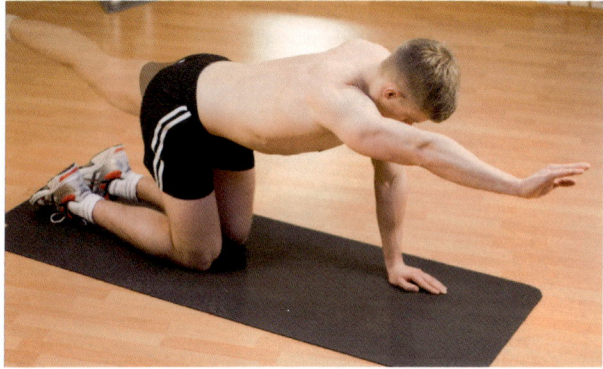

### Starting Position:

Kneel on all fours, with knees under hips and hands under shoulders. Make sure you keep a small, inward curve in your low back. Keep your neck long, your shoulder blades down and your elbows unlocked.

### Action:

Reach one arm forwards off the floor as far as control can be maintained through your pelvis and low back. Repeat with the other arm. Slide one foot along the floor away from the body. Continue to reach and raise the leg off the floor as far as control can be maintained. Repeat with the other leg.

**Repeat alternating arms eight to 10 times and repeat with the legs**

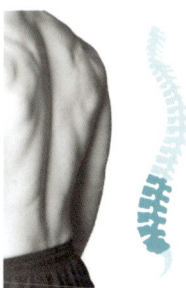

### Watch points
- Keep you neck long and deep abdominals activated throughout.
- Keep the correct curvature throughout the spine during the exercise.
- Lengthen and raise the leg by activating the buttocks Imagine a glass of water on your back throughout the exercise

THE BACK PAIN PERSONAL HEALTH PLAN    89

## LEVEL 1 — LOW BACK STRENGTHENING

# BRIDGING

**Aim:** To improve flexibility and stability of the spine

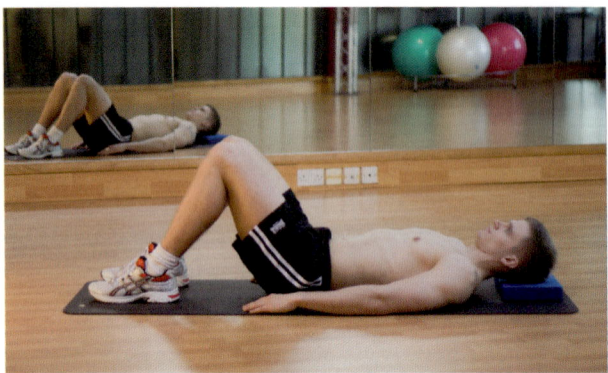
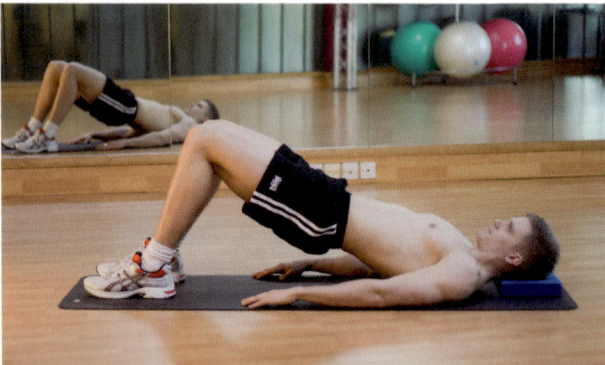

## Starting Position:

Lie on your back on a mat or the carpet. Place a small, flat cushion or book under your head. Bend your knees and keep your feet straight and in line with your hips. Keep your chest and ribcage relaxed and your chin gently tucked in.

## Action:

Activate your deep spinal muscles and gently roll your lower back into the mat. Scoop your tailbone upwards and continue to peel your spine off the mat, vertebra by vertebra, until you are resting on your shoulder blades. Achieve this by squeezing your buttocks during elevation. Lower one vertebra at a time onto the mat, beginning with the highest and finishing with your tailbone.

**Repeat eight to 10 times**

### Watch points
- Keep your deep abdominals activated throughout.
- Keep your neck long and relaxed.
- Relax your ribcage and do not push your chest forwards.
- Work through the buttocks not through the hamstrings.

**Variations:** Gently squeeze a towel or cushion between your knees.

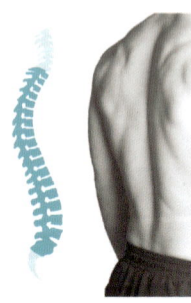

LOW BACK STRENGTHENING  LEVEL 1

# SIDE-LYING LEG RAISE

Aim: To strengthen the buttocks and low back

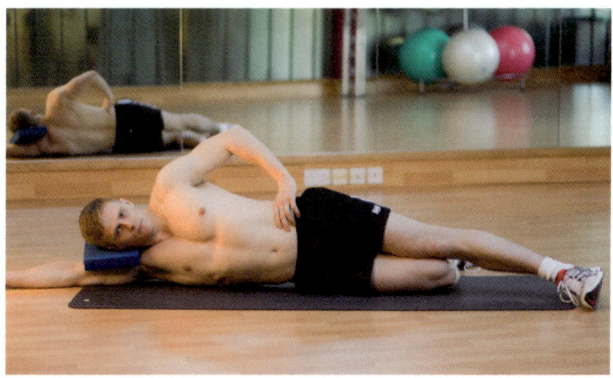
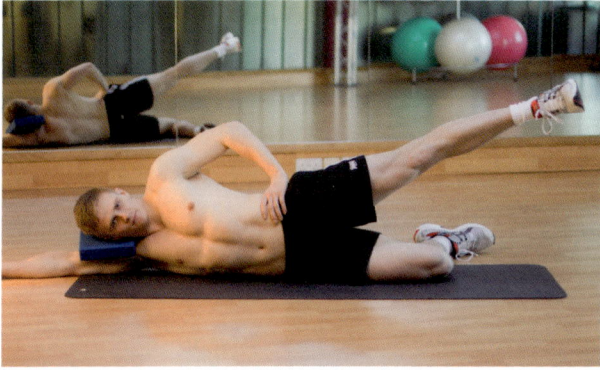

### Starting Position:

Lie on your side with your bottom knee bent to 90 degrees and your top leg straight and in line with your spine. Keep your hips stacked on top of each other. Gently press with your fingers into the muscle of your upper buttock (in the area where the back pocket of your trousers would be) to keep your hip forward.

### Action:

Raise the top leg towards the ceiling. Do not let your pelvis roll backwards. Slowly lower to the starting position.

**Repeat eight to 10 times on one side, then change sides and repeat.**

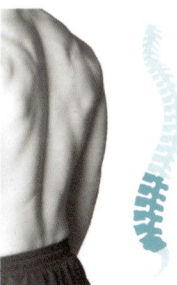

**Watch points**
- Keep your top hip forward throughout the exercise
- Raise your leg in line with your spine.
- Keep your deep abdominals activated throughout.
- Use a mirror to check your alignment during the exercise.

THE BACK PAIN PERSONAL HEALTH PLAN

**LEVEL 2**

# LOW BACK STRENGTHENING

Now that you have a solid foundation around your spine by achieving Level 1, you can challenge your back and build further strength and control with these advanced exercises.

### Benefits of Low Back Strengthening Level 2
- ✓ Increased strength and endurance in your abdominals and low back
- ✓ Improved posture
- ✓ Confidence to return to your previous sport or activities
- ✓ Improved body awareness and muscle activation

## The Routine

- Start the Level 2 exercises, follow each exercise instruction and gradually increase to the recommended amount of repetitions.
- Repeat Level 2 exercises every other day, in order to allow your muscles to fully recover from their workout.
- Between exercises, try to rest for no longer than five seconds.
- Keep each motion slow and controlled.
- Remember to retain the abdominal breathing throughout the exercises.

LOW BACK STRENGTHENING **LEVEL 2**

# BRIDGING

**Aim:** To improve flexibility and stability of the spine

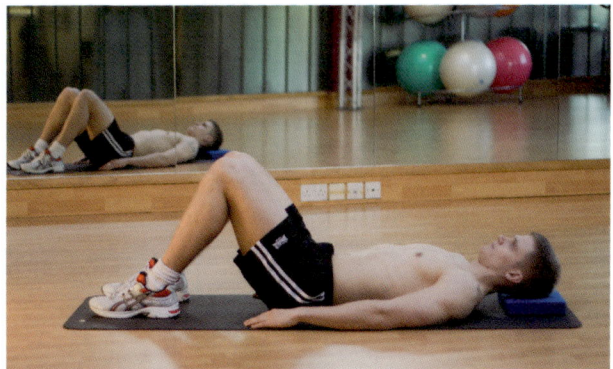

## Starting Position:

Lie on your back on a mat or the carpet. Place a small, flat cushion or book under your head. Bend your knees and keep your feet straight and in line with your hips. Keep your chest and ribcage relaxed and your chin gently tucked in.

## Action:

After raising the spine off the floor, straighten one leg and slowly lower it, just as you did for Bridging Level 1.

**Repeat, alternating legs, eight to 10 times.**

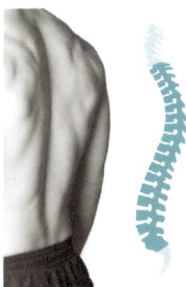

### Watch points
- Keep your deep abdominals activated throughout
- Keep both sides of your pelvis level and do not allow one side to dip whilst straightening one knee

THE BACK PAIN PERSONAL HEALTH PLAN   93

# LEVEL 2

## LOW BACK STRENGTHENING
## SWIMMING

**Aim:** To strengthen the low back and buttocks

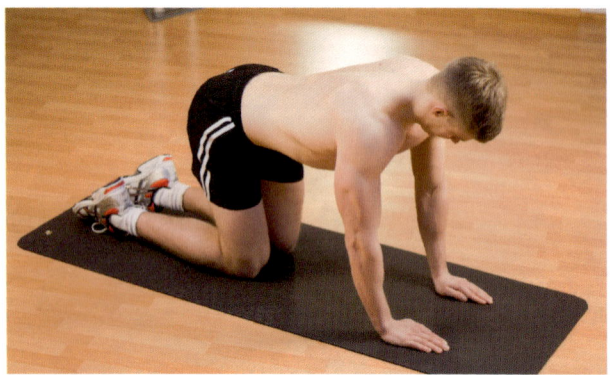
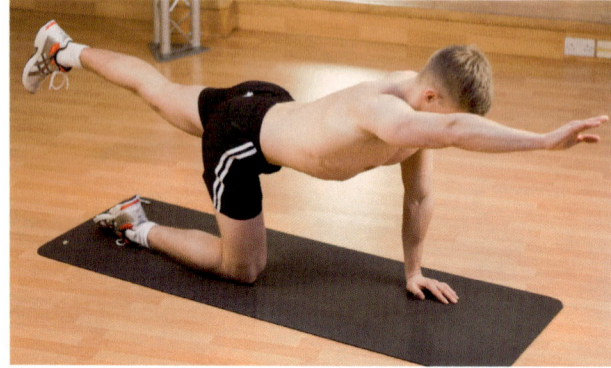

### Starting Position:

Kneel on all fours, with knees under hips and hands under shoulders. Make sure you keep a small, inward curve in your low back. Keep your neck long, your shoulder blades down and your elbows unlocked.

### Action:

Reach one arm forwards off the floor whilst simultaneously sliding the opposite foot along the floor away from the body. Continue to reach and raise the leg off the floor as far as control can be maintained through your pelvis and low back.

**Repeat alternating arms and legs eight to 10 times.**

### Watch points
- Keep you neck long and deep abdominals activated throughout.
- Keep the correct curvature throughout the spine during the exercise.
- Lengthen and raise the leg by activating the buttocks.
- Imagine a glass of water on your back throughout the exercise.

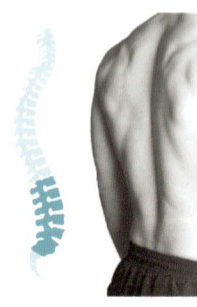

LOW BACK STRENGTHENING  LEVEL 2

# PLANK EXERCISE

**Aim:** To strengthen and stabilise the low back

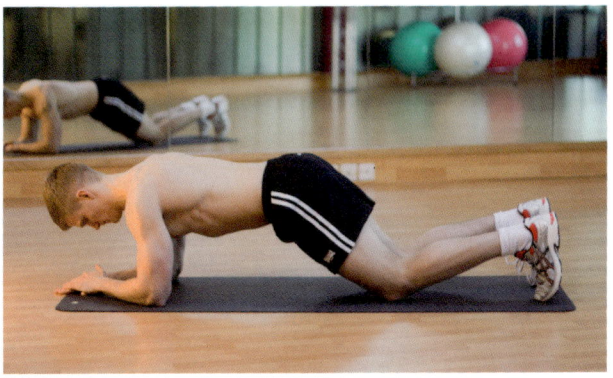 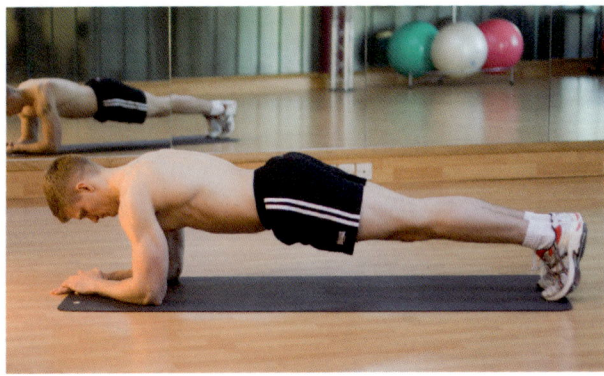

## Starting Position:

Lie on your front propped up on your forearms, knees and toes.

## Action:

Lift your pelvis and knees off the floor, creating a horizontal line from shoulders to ankles.
Hold for five to 10 seconds.

**Repeat eight to 10 times.**

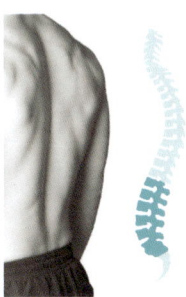

**Watch points**
- Do not allow your low back to dip down during the exercise.
- Keep your deep abdominals activated throughout.
- Use a mirror to check your alignment during the exercise.

**Variations:** If you find this difficult start by supporting your weight through the knees not the feet, over time gradually take your knees backwards

**LEVEL 2**

LOW BACK STRENGTHENING

# SIDE PLANK EXERCISE

**Aim:** To strengthen and stabilise the low back

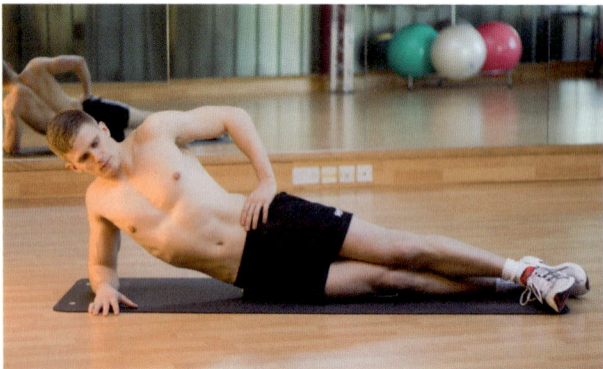 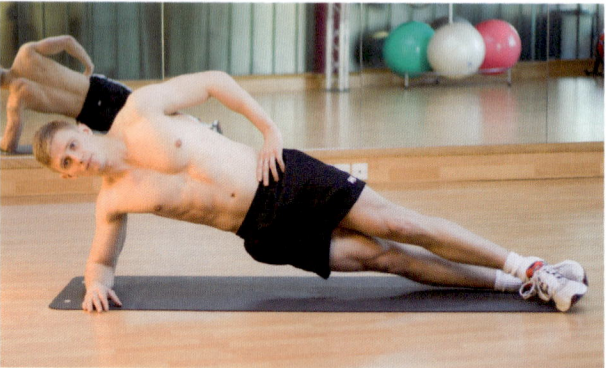

## Starting Position:

Lie on your side supporting your upper body weight on your forearm and keeping a straight line from your shoulders to your ankles. Keep your neck long and shoulder blades down.

## Action:

Raise your pelvis upwards until you achieve a straight line from shoulders to ankles. Hold for five to 10 seconds.

**Repeat eight to 10 times.**

### Watch points
- Keep your pelvis forward throughout the exercise.
- Keep your deep abdominals activated throughout.
- Use a mirror to check your alignment during the exercise.

**Variations:** If you find this difficult start by supporting your weight through the knee not the feet.

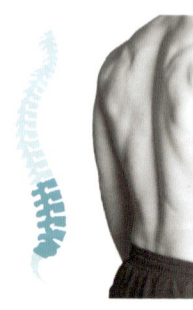

96   THE BACK PAIN PERSONAL HEALTH PLAN

# BUTTOCK & LEG STRETCHES

So far, your exercise programme has concentrated on strengthening and stretching your back and neck. But if you suffer from low back pain and leg pain, the tightness of your buttock and leg muscles may well be a contributing factor to your pain.

These exercises will help you to recognise tightness in specific muscles of the buttocks or legs and guide you in improving the flexibility of these muscles

It takes weeks or months to see the benefits of regular stretching, so patience and perseverance are important factors in your improvement regime.

### Benefits of Buttock and Leg Stretches
- ✓ Improved flexibility of the leg muscles
- ✓ Less tension on the low back and sciatic nerve
- ✓ Improved posture
- ✓ Less discomfort in the legs and low back
- ✓ Greater ease in undertaking daily tasks

## The Routine
- Hold each stretch for 20-30 seconds whilst taking deep abdominal breathes
- Repeat each stretch two to three times daily.

BUTTOCK AND LEG STRETCHES

# KNEELING QUAD STRETCH

**Aim:** To stretch the thigh and hip muscles

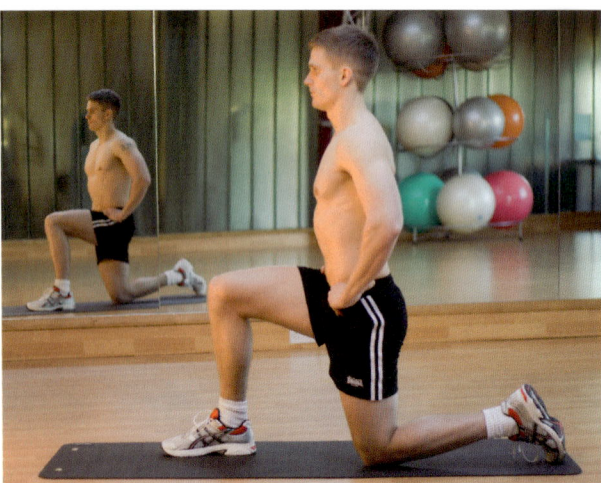 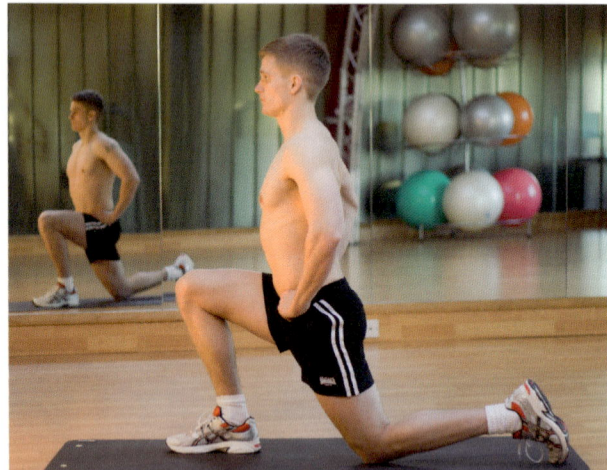

## Technique

Kneel on one foot and the other knee. If needed, hold onto something to keep your balance. Keep your back straight and push your hips forward. Feel for a stretch in the front of the hip and thigh.
Hold for 20-30 seconds whilst taking deep breaths.

**Repeat two to three times.**

### Watch points
- Place a pillow under your knee if needed for comfort.
- Keep your hips square throughout the exercise.
- Only stretch as far as is comfortable.

BUTTOCK AND LEG STRETCHE

# STANDING HAMSTRING STRETCH

**Aim:** To stretch and lengthen the hamstring muscles

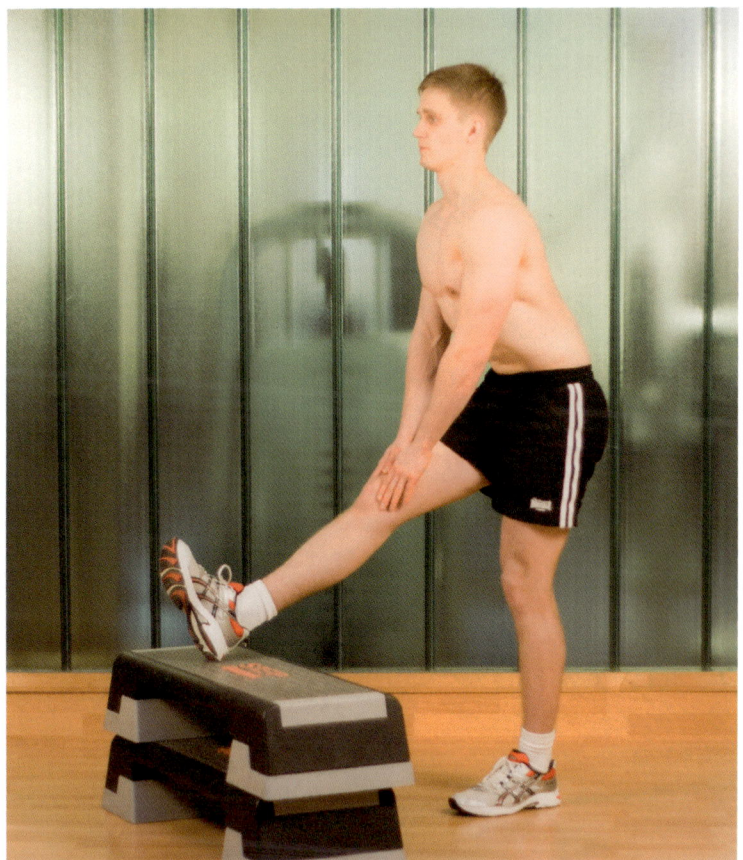

## Technique

Stand upright and raise one leg on to an object. Keep that leg straight and your toes pointing straight up. Lean forward whilst keeping your back straight. Hold for 20-30 seconds whilst taking deep breaths.

**Repeat two to three times.**

### Watch points
- Only stretch as far as is comfortable.
- Your low back should not arch at any time.

BUTTOCK AND LEG STRETCHES

# STANDING QUAD STRETCH

**Aim:** To stretch and lengthen the thigh muscles

## Technique

Stand upright whilst balancing on one leg. Hold onto something for balance. Pull your other foot up behind your buttocks and keep your knees together whilst tucking your tailbone under and pushing your hips forward.
Hold for 20-30 seconds whilst taking deep breaths.

**Repeat two to three times.**

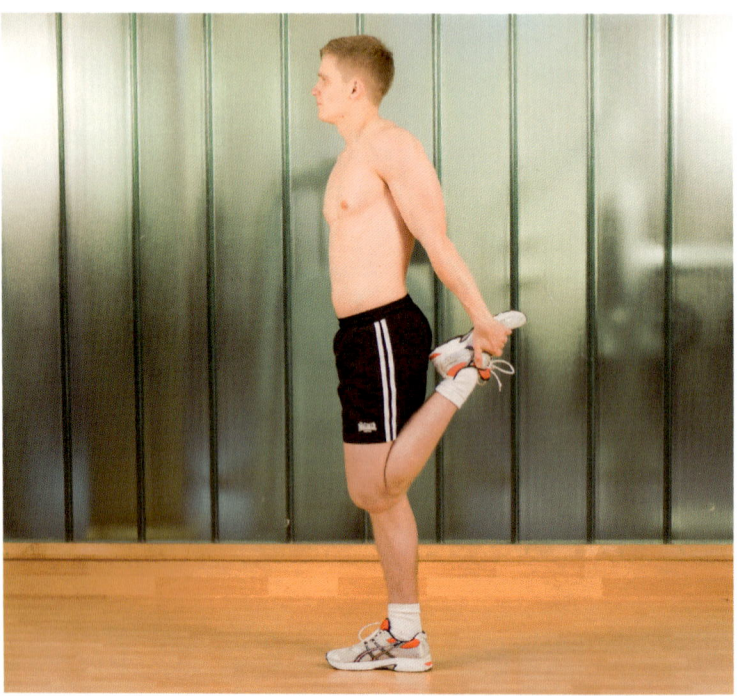

### Watch points
- If you suffer from knee pain, avoid this stretch.
- Keep your knees together throughout the exercise.
- Do not lean forwards.
- Only stretch as far as is comfortable
- Hold onto the bottom of your trousers or hold onto a towel around your ankle to make the stretch easier

BUTTOCK AND LEG STRETCHE

# LEANING CALF STRETCH

**Aim:** To stretch and lengthen the calf muscles

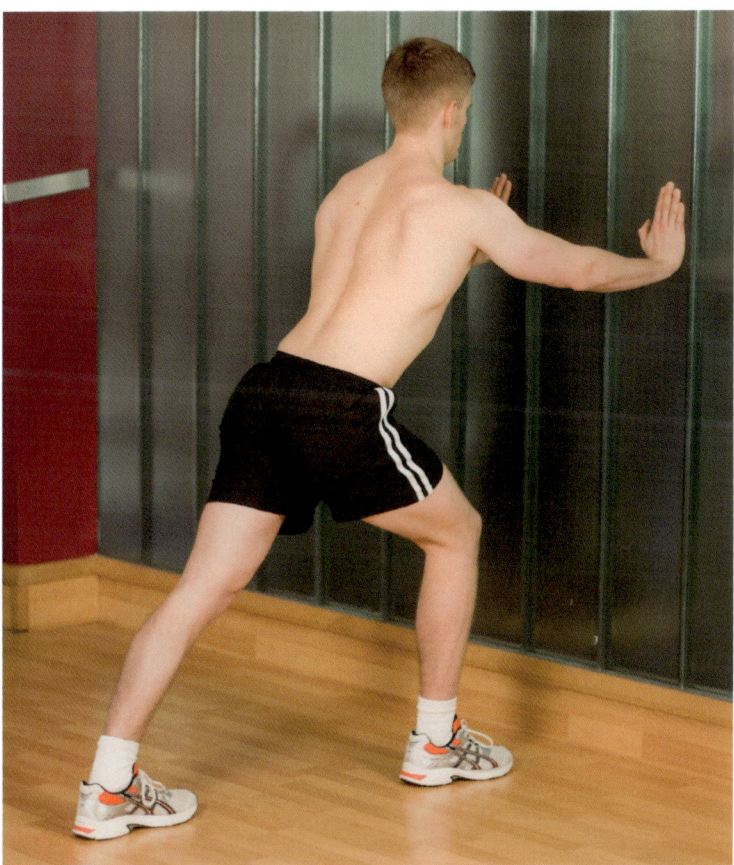

## Technique

Stand upright and lean against a wall. Place one foot as far from the wall as is comfortable and make sure that both toes are facing forward and your heel is on the ground. Keep your back leg straight and lean forward.
Hold for 20-30 seconds whilst taking deep breaths.

**Repeat two to three times.**

### Watch points
- Make sure the toes and foot of the back leg are facing forward.
- Only stretch as far as is comfortable.

BUTTOCK AND LEG STRETCHES

# LYING CROSS KNEE PULL UP STRETCH

**Aim:** To stretch and lengthen the buttocks

## Technique

Lie on your back and cross on leg over the other. Bring your foot up to your opposite knee and with your opposite arm pull your raised knee up towards your chest. Hold for 20-30 seconds while taking deep breathes.

**Repeat two to three times.**

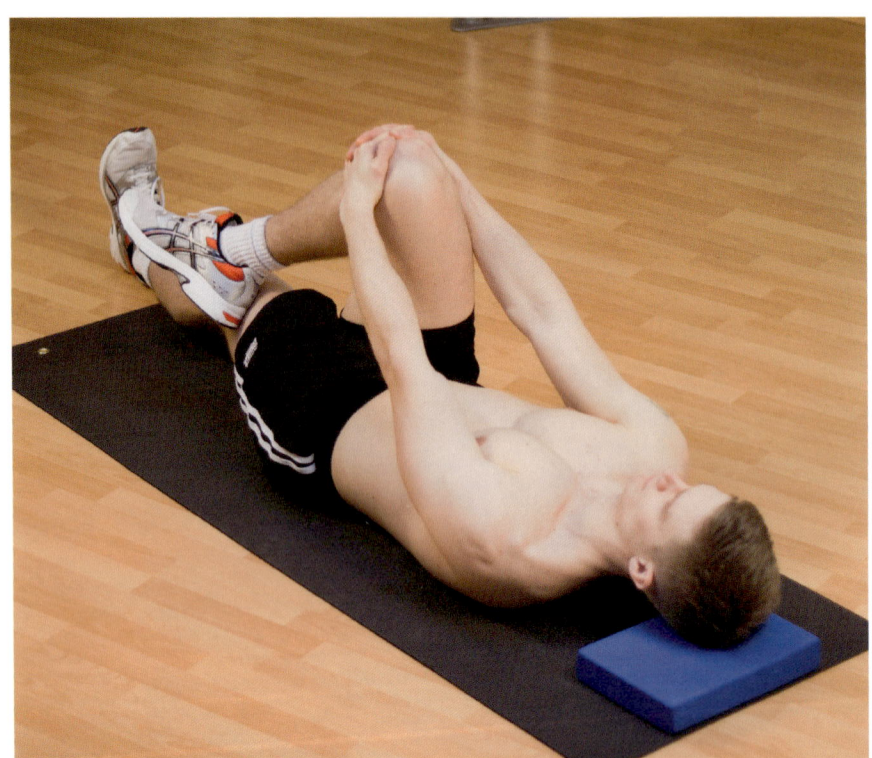

### Watch points
- Keep both shoulders on the ground.
- Only stretch as far as is comfortable.

BUTTOCK AND LEG STRETCHE

# LYING DEEP GLUTEAL STRETCH

**Aim:** To stretch and lengthen the piriformis muscle

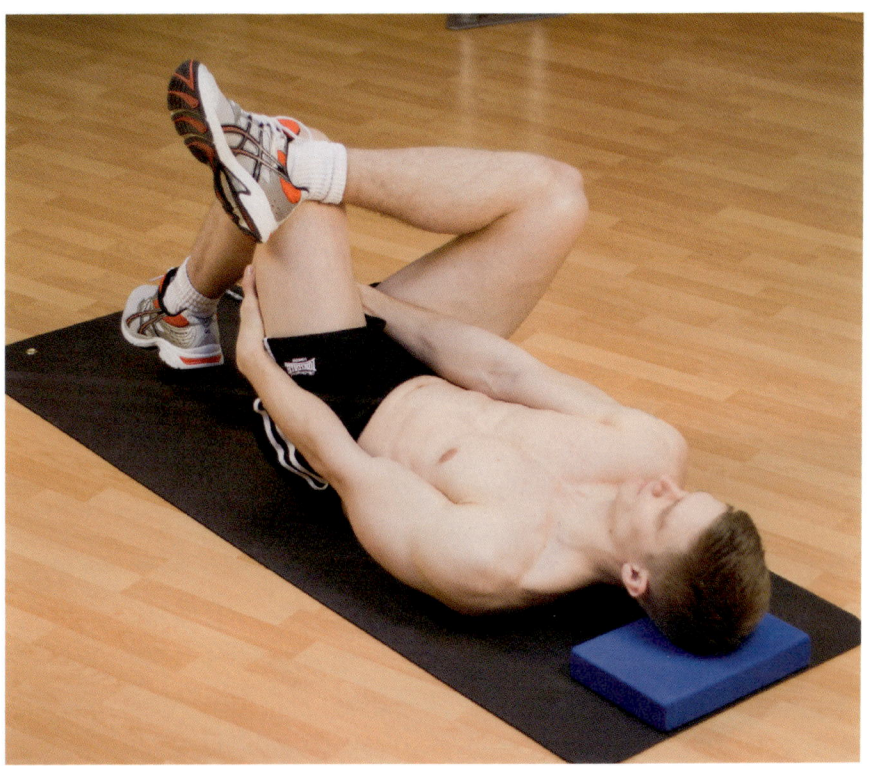

## Technique

Lie on your back and bend one leg. Raise the other foot up onto the other leg and rest it on your thigh. Then reach forward holding onto your knee and pull towards you. Keep your tailbone on the floor throughout and your pelvis square. You should feel the stretch in the buttock of the leg resting on the other knee. This is a difficult stretch so use a towel around the knee if you are unable to perform the stretch
Hold for 20-30 seconds while taking deep breaths.

**Repeat two to three times.**

### Watch points
- Only stretch as far as is comfortable.
- Do not let your tailbone tuck under you.
- Keep your pelvis square.

# NECK EXERCISES

If you suffer from pain or muscular tension in the neck or shoulders then this is the section for you! You will learn how to identify your muscle tightness and how to stretch these areas. You will also learn strengthening exercises for the neck and shoulder blades to take the strain away from these painful areas.

## Benefits of the Neck Exercises
- ✓ Improved posture
- ✓ Less discomfort in your neck and shoulders
- ✓ Less muscle tension around your shoulder blades
- ✓ Increased strength and endurance in your neck and shoulders

## The Routine

- Practise the stretches to identify your areas of muscle tightness, and do these exercises as recommended daily.
- Work through the strengthening section and perform this routine every day.
- Follow each exercise instruction and gradually increase to the recommended amount
- Keep each motion slow and controlled
- Remember to maintain abdominal breathing throughout the exercises.

NECK STRETCHING EXERCISES

# TENSION RELIEVING NECK STRETCH

**Aim:** To reduce tension and stretch the neck

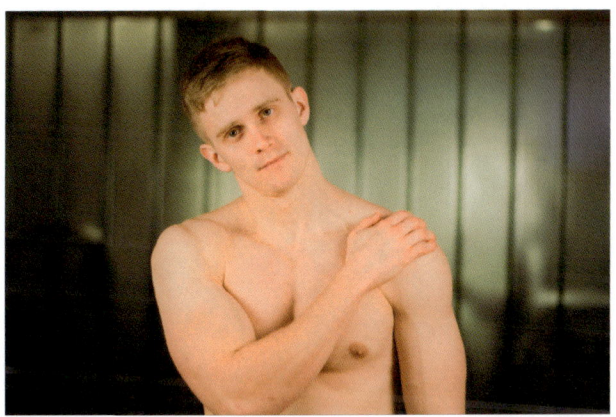

## Starting Position:

Sit in a chair whilst keeping your shoulder blades down and your neck long. Place your left hand on your right shoulder.

## Action:

Lower your left ear towards your left shoulder. Only stretch as far as is comfortable.
Hold for 20-30 seconds whilst taking deep abdominal breathes.

Repeat on alternating sides, 2 or 3 times each.

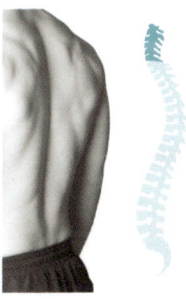

### Watch points
- Use your hand to stop your shoulder from raising up during the exercise.
- Keep your neck long and shoulder blades down throughout.

**Variations:** Experiment during the stretch by rotating the head slightly to target tight areas within the muscle.
To help keep the shoulder down, hold underneath the chair or interlock the fingers behind the back.

NECK STRETCHING EXERCISES

# FORWARD FLEXION NECK STRETCH

**Aim:** Forward Flexion Neck Stretch

## Technique

Stand or sit upright. Now, slowly draw the chin inwards and then let your chin fall towards your chest. Keep your shoulder blades down and relaxed throughout. Hold for 20-30 seconds whilst taking deep breaths.

Repeat two to three times.

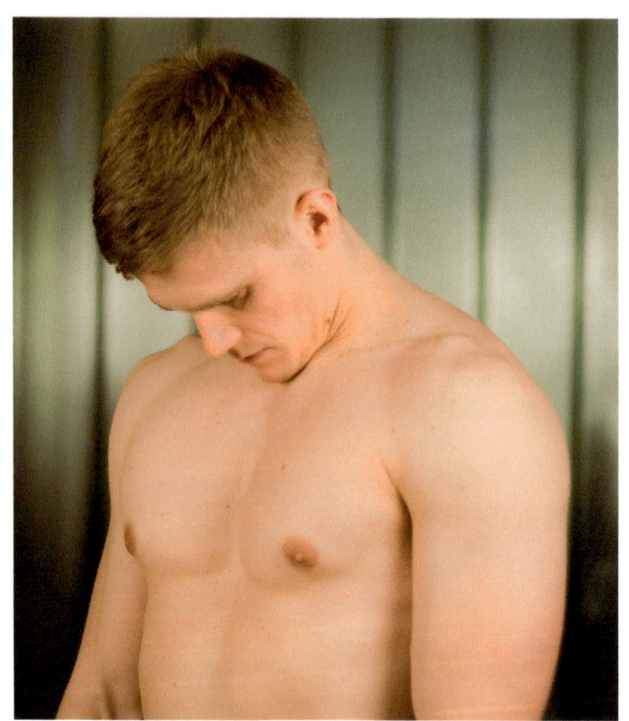

Watch points
- Do not overstretch by forcing your head down: let the weight of your head provide the necessary pressure
- Only stretch as far as is comfortable

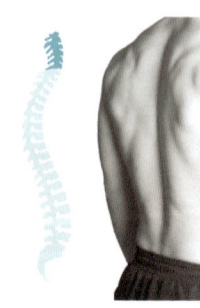

106    THE BACK PAIN PERSONAL HEALTH PLAN

NECK STRETCHING EXERCISES

# NECK ROTATION STRETCH

**Aim:** To stretch the neck muscles and mobilise the joints in the neck and upper back

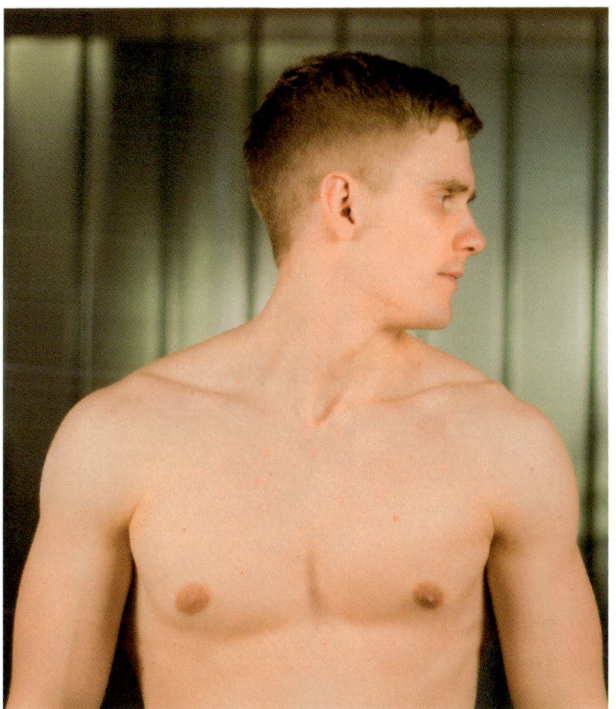

## Technique

Stand or sit upright. Keep your shoulder blades down and relaxed. Slowly rotate your chin towards your opposite shoulder. Hold for 20-30 seconds whilst taking deep breaths.

**Repeat two to three times.**

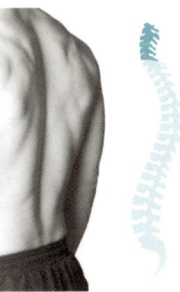

### Watch points
- Keep your head up and do not let your chin fall towards your chest or shoulders
- Only stretch as far as is comfortable.

NECK STRETCHING EXERCISES

# CHEST STRETCH

**Aim:** To improve posture and stretch the chest and upper shoulders

## Starting Position:

Stand with your spine in correct alignment and your hands on your hips. Keep your neck long and shoulder blades down throughout the exercise.

## Action:

Slowly pull your shoulders back and your elbows towards each other. Hold for 20-30 seconds. Slowly return to the starting position.

**Repeat eight to 10 times.**

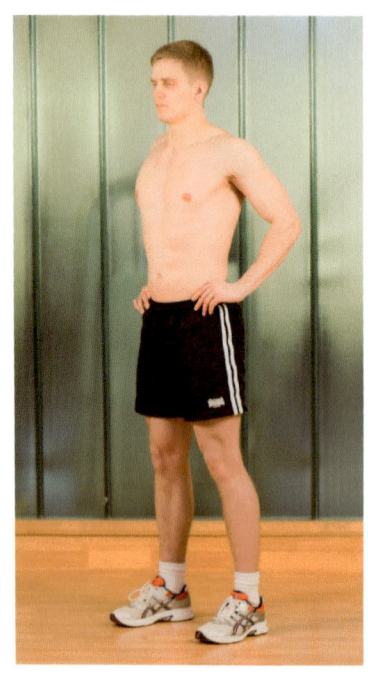
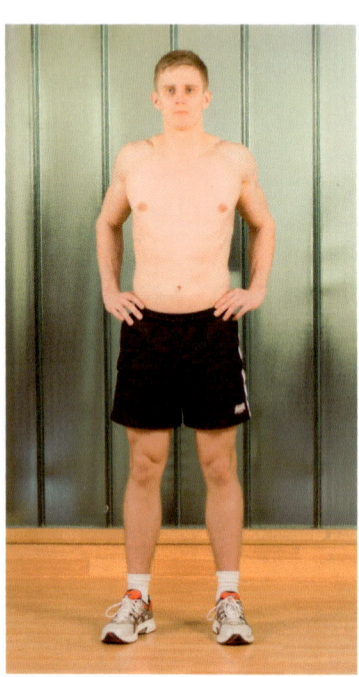

### Watch points
- Do not arch your back during the exercise.
- Keep your neck long.
- Only stretch as far as is comfortable.

**Variations:** To progress the stretch, interlock your fingers behind your back, pull your shoulders back and lift your hands away from you.

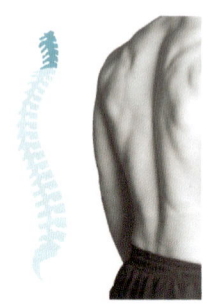

108    THE BACK PAIN PERSONAL HEALTH PLAN

NECK STRENGTHENING EXERCISES

# CHIN TUCKS

Aim: To reduce tension in the neck and strengthen the deep postural muscles

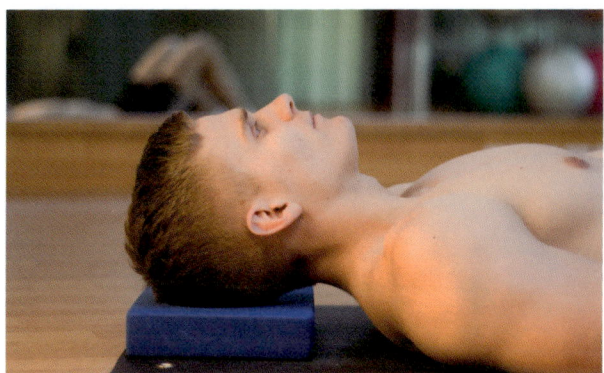 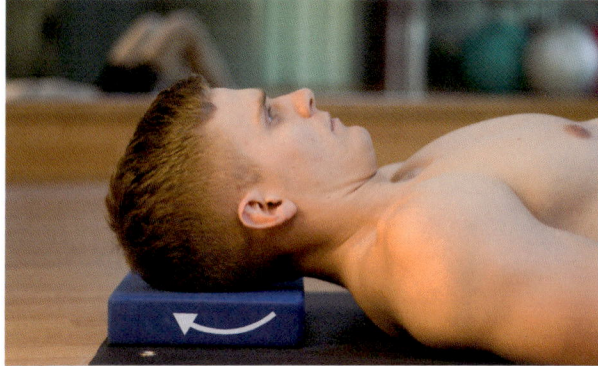

## Starting Position:

Lie on your back on a mat or the carpet. Place a small, flat cushion or book under your head. Bend your knees and keep your feet straight and in line with your hips. Keep your chest and ribcage relaxed and your chin gently tucked in.

## Action:

Gently lengthen the back of the neck feeling the chin slowly draw inwards. Hold for eight to 10 breaths.

**Repeat up to 10 times.**

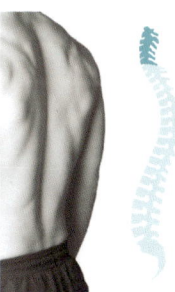

### Watch points
- Make sure your head remains on the floor.
- Keep the large muscles on the front of the neck relaxed throughout.
- Ensure your movements are slow and smooth, not fast and jerky.
- Make sure your shoulders and chest remain relaxed.

**Variations:** After drawing the neck inwards, roll your neck slowly to the side. Never move into pain. Slowly return and repeat to the other side.

NECK STRENGTHENING EXERCISES

# SHOULDER BLADE & NECK STRENGTHENING

**Aim:** To strengthen the postural muscles around the neck and shoulder blades and reduce muscle tension.

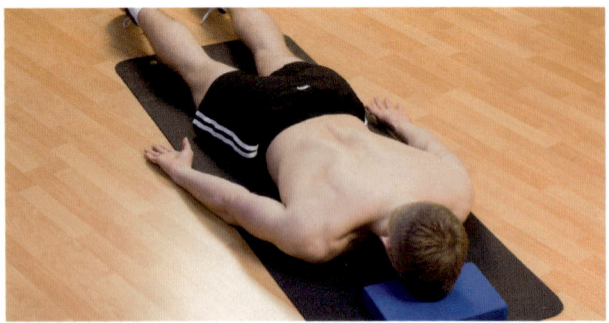
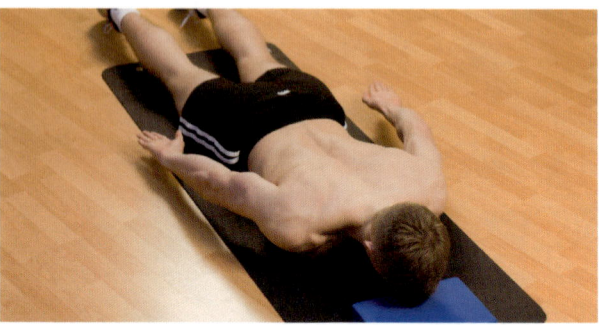

## Starting Position:

Lie on your front with a small, folded towel or flat cushion under your forehead. Keep your neck long, as you do in the "Chin Tucks" exercise.

## Action:

Slide your shoulder blades down into your back away from your ears. Hold for three to five breaths. Relax the shoulder blades to the starting position. The head remains down and the neck long.

**Repeat eight to 10 times.**

Watch points
- Do not squeeze your arms into your sides. Imagine you are holding a ripe peach between your arm and your body.
- Do not allow your low back to arch. Use a folded towel under your stomach to avoid this.
- Stop if you feel any pain in your neck or back.

**Variations:** To progress the exercise further, try hovering your hands one inch from the floor after sliding your shoulder blades down.
When you are comfortable with the previous variation, you can progress to simultaneously hovering the forehead one inch off the towel, keeping your neck long.

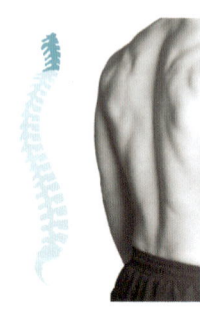

110  THE BACK PAIN PERSONAL HEALTH PLAN

# GENERAL AEROBIC EXERCISE PROGRAMME

This section is designed to start you off with a simple workout, consisting of straightforward aerobic exercises. This will build up your confidence and encourage you to return to the activities you enjoy. Increased activity will strengthen your back, help you sleep better at night, and have more energy during the day.

### Benefits of the General Aerobic Exercise Programme
- ✓ Strengthens your entire body
- ✓ Lowers blood pressure
- ✓ Helps decrease stress
- ✓ Burn calories and speed up your metabolism

Slowly build up the time you spend doing aerobic exercise each week. Below are some exercise ideas, which you might enjoy.

- A brisk walk
- Cycling
- Swimming
- An elliptical machine in the gym
- An exercise class, such as Pilates or yoga

GENERAL AEROBIC EXERCISE PROGRAMME

# SQUAT

Aim: A great overall exercise to increase flexibility and strength to the spine and leg muscles

## Starting Position:

Stand with your feet shoulder-width apart and feet facing forwards. Hold your hands straight out in front of you.

## Action:

Bend your knees, and as you sink, sit back as if you were heading for a chair. Push your chest forward and keep your head up and looking straight in front of you. Do not let your knees push forward and aim to keep equal weight between the front and back of your feet. Go down as far as is comfortable, aiming so your thighs are parallel to the floor. Slowly rise back to the starting position.

Repeat eight to 10 times.

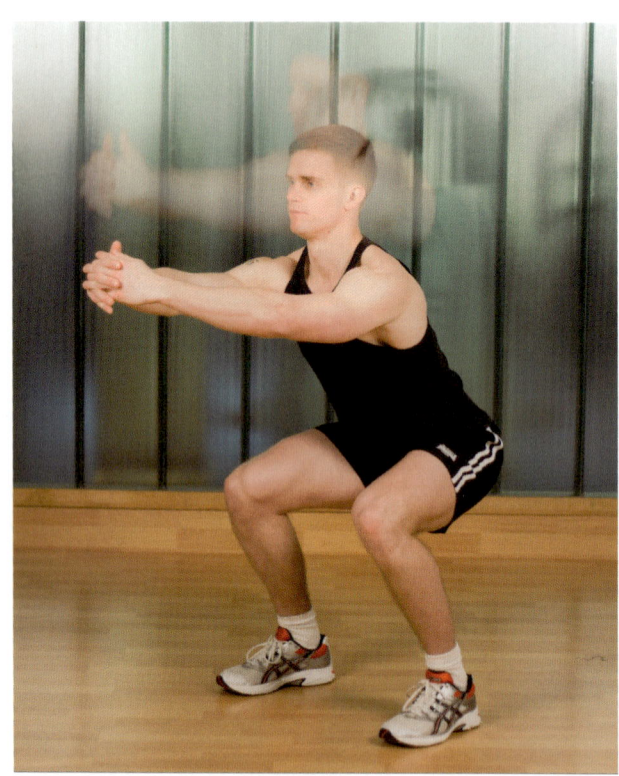

### Watch points
- Always keep your heels on the floor and your spine in alignment.
- It may take weeks till your thighs are parallel to the floor, but make this one of your goals. This will increase your flexibility and strength to the spine and legs.
- Never bounce in the squat position.

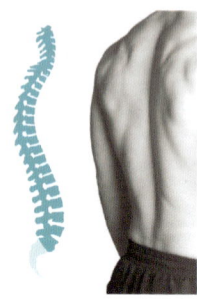

GENERAL AEROBIC EXERCISE PROGRAMME

# WALL PRESS UPS

**Aim:** To strengthen the upper body and spine

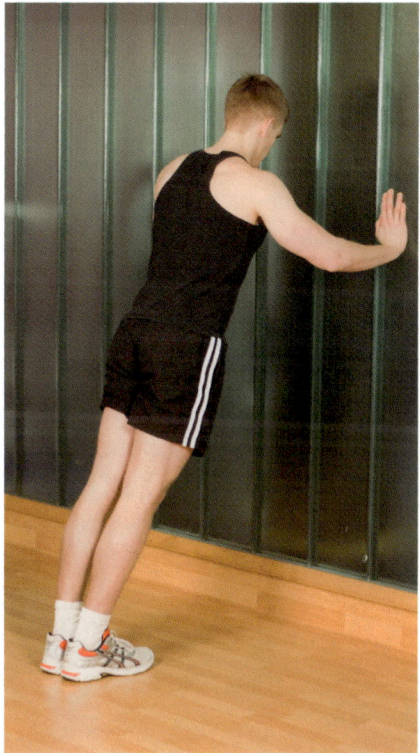
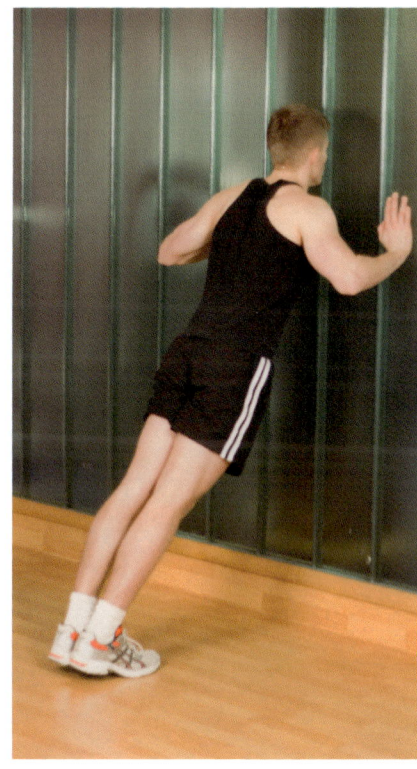

## Starting Position:

Place your hands on a wall at shoulder height and just wider than shoulder-width apart. Your feet should be shoulder-width apart and positioned some distance away from the wall.

## Action:

Keeping your chest and head up, take your chest down towards the wall, whilst keeping your legs in line with your spine. Slowly return to the starting position.

**Repeat eight to 10 times.**

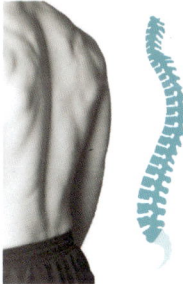

### Watch points
- Keep your deep abdominals contracted throughout
- Do not bend from the waist
- To make the exercise harder, move your feet further away from the wall

THE BACK PAIN PERSONAL HEALTH PLAN

GENERAL AEROBIC EXERCISE PROGRAMME

# STAR-SHAPED SIDE STEPS

**Aim:** A great aerobic exercise for the entire body

## Starting Position:
Stand upright, with your arms at your sides.

## Action:
Step sideways and in the same movement raise up the arms. Repeat five times on one side and then five times on the alternate side.

**Repeat the sequence eight to 10 times on both sides.**

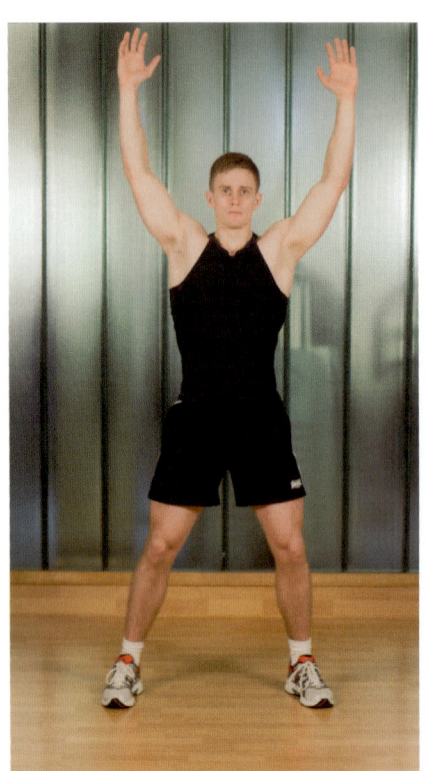
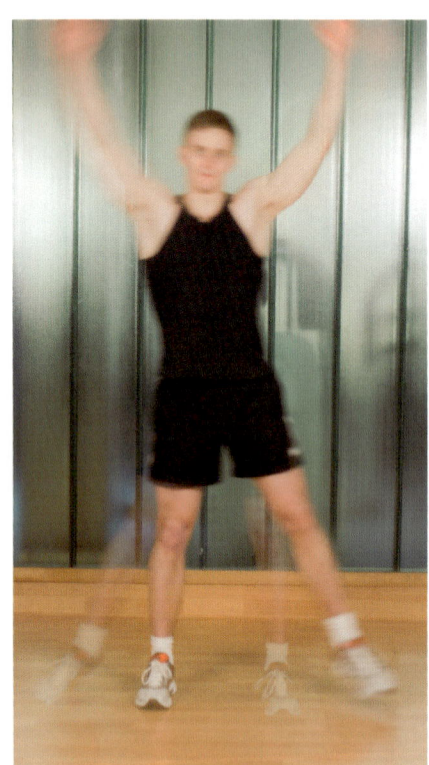

### Watch points
- Keep your deep abdominals contracted throughout.
- If you have shoulder problems, use an alternate arm exercise.

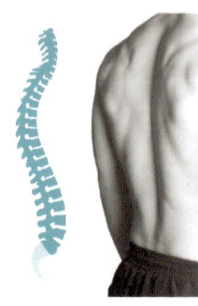

114   THE BACK PAIN PERSONAL HEALTH PLAN

GENERAL AEROBIC EXERCISE PROGRAMME

# HIGH KNEES

Aim: To improve balance and exercise the arms and legs

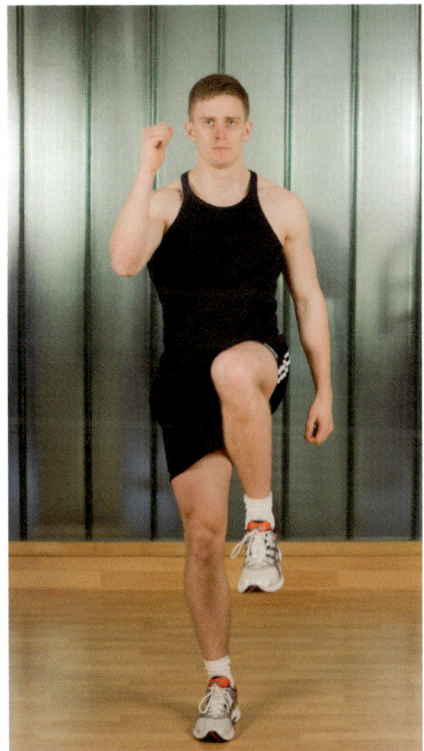
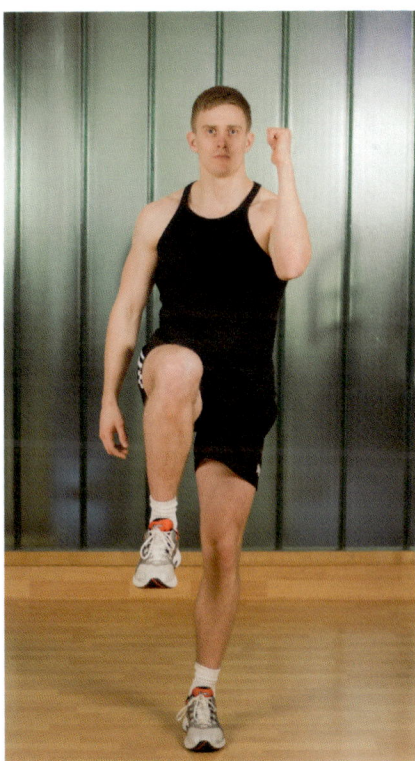

## Starting Position:

Stand upright, with your arms at your sides.

## Action:

Bring one knee up to the horizontal position whilst simultaneously bending the elbows into a bicep curl. Next, lower the leg and arms to the starting position, and then repeat for the other leg.

Repeat 10–20 times with each leg.

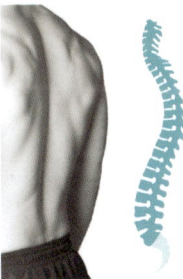

### Watch points
- Keep your deep abdominals contracted throughout.
- Keep the pelvis and spine still throughout the exercise.
- Add hand weights to increase difficulty.

GENERAL AEROBIC EXERCISE PROGRAMME

# HEEL TO BOTTOM

**Aim:** To improve balance, spinal control and stretch the front of the legs.

## Starting Position:

Stand upright, with your arms at your sides.

## Action:

Bend one knee bringing the heel as far as possible up to the buttock, whilst simultaneously bending your elbows into a bicep curl. Return to the starting position and repeat for the other leg.

Repeat 10–20 times with each leg.

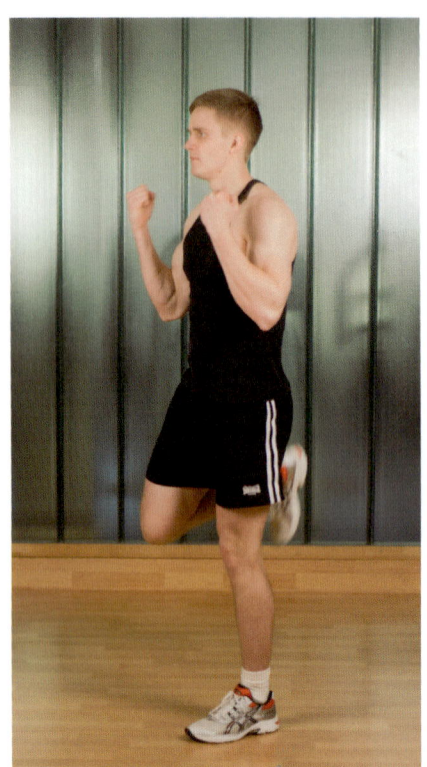
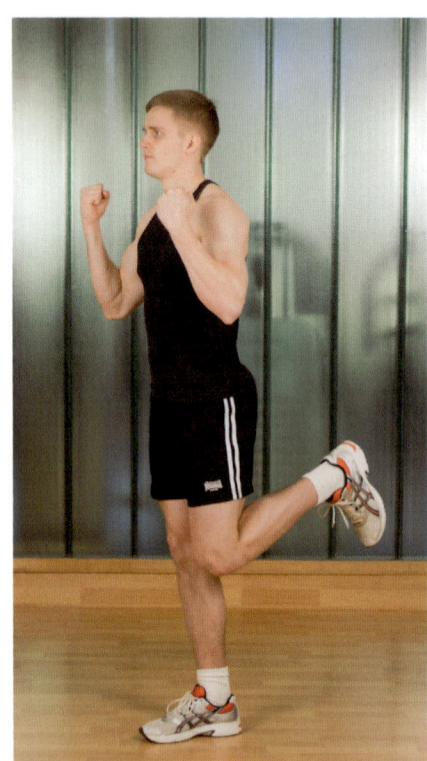

### Watch points
- Keep your deep abdominals contracted throughout.
- Only stretch as far as is comfortable.
- Keep the pelvis and spine still throughout the exercise.

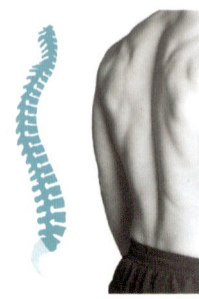

GENERAL AEROBIC EXERCISE PROGRAMME

# STEP UPS

**Aim:** To improve aerobic endurance and strengthen the back.

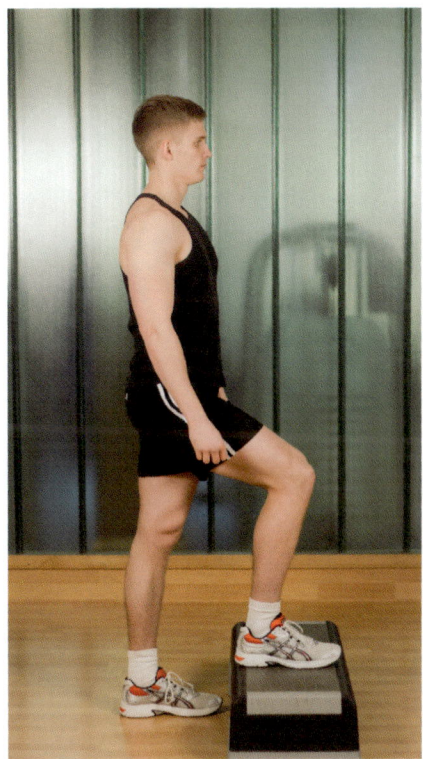
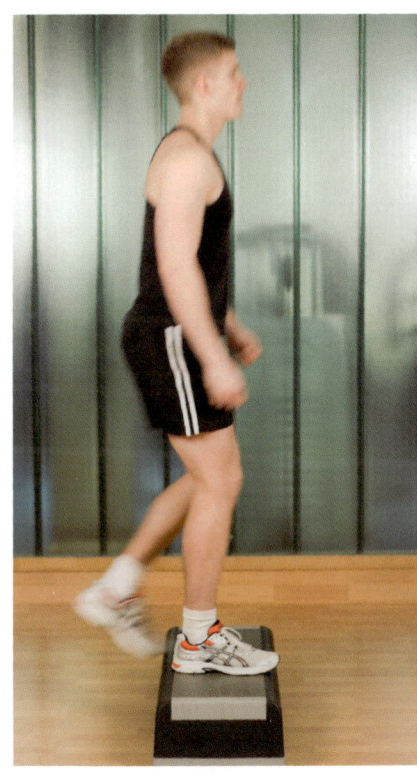

## Starting Position:

Standing facing a step. If no step is available, use a few large books stacked against a wall.

## Action:

Step up with one leg onto the step, followed by the other leg. Now step down using the leading leg, and then bring the other leg down to the starting position.

> Step up and down 10-20 times leading with one leg, then change legs and repeat.

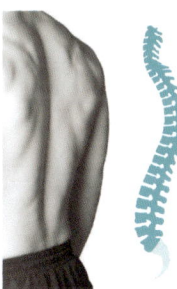

**Watch points**
- The slower you raise and lower the leg, the harder the muscles work.
- Keep the knee over the toes when stepping up.
- Keep your deep abdominals contracted throughout.
- Keep the pelvis and spine still throughout the exercise.

# MY ACTION PLAN

**To improve my health and wellbeing this is what I would like to achieve** (set short-, medium- and long-term goals):

| | |
|---|---|
| Short term: | Target date: |
| Medium term: | Target date: |
| Long term: | Target date: |

**This is what I will do to help achieve these goals:**

Include skills 1-5 of the programme.

**This is the support I need to help me to achieve my goals:**

To include the support I require and who I require it from.

**What to do in the event of a flare up:**

Include skills 1-5 of the programme.

# MY ACTION PLAN

| **Additional help and support** | |
|---|---|
| I would like access to a support programme to help me manage my back pain needs? | ☐ Yes<br>☐ No |

**Other information relevant to my needs**

| **Questions I would like to ask my health professional at my next appointment:** |
|---|
| |

| **Additional information relating to clinics, letters and records of consultation:** |
|---|
| |

# THE 5 SKILLS OF THE PHP

| Skill | Actions |
|---|---|
| **Skill 1:** Mindset | e.g. Keep positive and expect recovery |
| **Skill 2:** Lifestyle Management | e.g. Improve posture, correct lifting technique |
| **Skill 3:** Pain Management | e.g. Pacing, heat, self massage |
| **Skill 4:** Exercise | e.g. develop fitness programme |
| **Skill 5:** Healthy Living | e.g. quit smoking, manage weight |

# THE 5 SKILLS OF THE PHP

| Skill | Goals |
|---|---|
| **Skill 1:** Mindset | Include short, medium and long term goals |
| **Skill 2:** Lifestyle Management | Include short, medium and long term goals |
| **Skill 3:** Pain Management | Include short, medium and long term goals |
| **Skill 4:** Exercise | Include short, medium and long term goals |
| **Skill 5:** Healthy Living | Include short, medium and long term goals |

# EXERCISE GLOSSARY

### Breathing exercises

- ☐ Breathing exercises **60**

### Muscle imbalance

- ☐ Lack of stretching **62**
- ☐ Sedentary lifestyle **62**
- ☐ Left- or right-handedness **63**

### Postual awareness

- ☐ Prolonged sitting postures **66**
- ☐ Uneven sitting postures **66**
- ☐ Standing posture **67**

### Postural strengthening

- ☐ Postural strengthening **68**

### Back pain treatments

- ☐ Cold treatment **70**
- ☐ Heat treatment **70**
- ☐ Soft tissue massage or self-massage **70**
- ☐ Bending and lifting advice **70**

### Low back stretches

- ☐ Knee to chest stretch **75**
- ☐ Cat stretch **76**
- ☐ Bottom to heels stretch **77**
- ☐ Knee rolls **78**
- ☐ Sciatic mobilising stretch **79**
- ☐ Back extensions **80**
- ☐ Standing side bends **81**
- ☐ Spine rotations **82**

# EXERCISE GLOSSARY

### Low back strengthening Level 1

- ☐ Deep abdominal strengthening 84
- ☐ Pelvic tilts 85
- ☐ Leg slides 86
- ☐ Knee drops 87
- ☐ Leg lifts 88
- ☐ Swimming 89
- ☐ Bridging 90
- ☐ Side-lying leg raise 91

### Low back strengthening Level 2

- ☐ Bridging 93
- ☐ Swimming 94
- ☐ Plank exercise 95
- ☐ Side plank exercise 96

### Buttock & leg stretches

- ☐ Kneeling quad stretch 98
- ☐ Standing hamstring stretch 99
- ☐ Standing quad stretch 100
- ☐ Leaning calf stretch 101
- ☐ Lying cross knee pull up stretch 102
- ☐ Lying deep gluteal stretch 103

### Neck exercises

- ☐ Tension relieving neck stretch 105
- ☐ Forward flexion neck stretch 106
- ☐ Neck rotation stretch 107
- ☐ Chest stretch 108
- ☐ Chin tucks 109
- ☐ Shoulder blade & neck strengthening 110

### General aerobic exercise programme

- ☐ Squat 112
- ☐ Wall press ups 113
- ☐ Star-shaped side steps 114
- ☐ High knees 115
- ☐ Heel to bottom 116
- ☐ Step ups 117

# ABOUT THE AUTHOR

Nick Sinfield MCSP, HPC is a Chartered Physiotherapist and Clinical Director at Therapy Programmes Limited. His health programmes have been featured in the national press and on BBC radio.

Nick is also the author of "Now I Can Bend My Back!" The Essential Guide to Back and Neck Pain. In 2011 he was a Finalist at the Chartered Society of Physiotherapy Congress.

The Back Pain Personal Health Plan was inspired from working with leading physiotherapists in the U.K., New Zealand and Australia. The programme was written with one purpose in mind; to return control to the person in pain. It has taken the very complex and multi-factorial problem of back pain, explained it, and provided the reader with information and knowledge to address the problem.

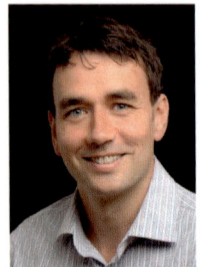

Nick Sinfield MCSP, HPC, APPI

# BIBLIOGRAPHY

Banyard P, Applying Psychology to Health, Hodder and Stoughton, 1996

Bean C A, The Better Back Book, Anaya Publishers, 1989

Butler D S, G Lorimer Moseley G L., Explain Pain, Noigroup Publications, 2003

Hage M, The Back Pain Book, Class Publishing, 2005

Keys, S., Back Sufferers Bible, Vermilion, 2000

Richardson C, Jull G, Hodges P, Hides J., Therapeutic Exercise for Spinal Segmental Stabilization in Low Back Pain, Churchill Livingstone, 1999

Robinson L, Fisher H, Massey P., Body Control Pilates Back Book, Pan Books, 2002

Sarno J E, Healing Back Pain, Warner Book, 1991

# SHORT-TERM GOALS

# LONG-TERM GOALS

# TESTIMONIALS

❝ This book has changed my whole outlook on where I see myself going in the future. I am now able to work again pain free and have returned to my boxing classes. I think differently about my back pain and will continue to follow your advice, many thanks! ❞

*Wayne Roberts, Builder, Bedfordshire*

❝ A very useful and handy book for back pain suffers. I will be recommending it to my patients. ❞

*Dr MC, medical doctor in the UK*

❝ I have been a patient of Nick's recently with low back pain. I found it increasingly painful to do minimal chores… Thanks to Nick with his exercise techniques my pain has been eliminated. ❞

*Dionne Gravestock, Amptill*

# TESTIMONIALS

" This self-help guide should be the answer to all those people who are confused by conflicting ideas about back pain. Clarity at last! Here is an attractive easy-to-access solution to many of the questions that are as aggravating as the pain and stiffness.

Nick has chosen to approach back problems through the Mind and how training it can help. This is in line with the latest research evidence and is the most effective way forward.

The next section looks at the factors involved in back activity including causes of pain and stiffness together with what helps and why. His exercise suggestions are graded and clearly illustrated with "watch points" for safe self-management.

I have trained many physiotherapists to run Back Fitness Groups and would like this book to be available to all groups. My hope is that the message of cognitive behavioural therapy and self-management with exercise will spread nationwide to so many back sufferers. This book is the best I have seen on the subject. I hope it will be widely available. "

*Anna Taylor MCSP, Physiotherapist and Course Founder of Back Fitness Group Workshops*

# TESTIMONIALS

" Having recently looked through referral rates at my practice...lower back and neck pain made up a large bulk of these referrals. It was, therefore, refreshing to see a book that I could easily read that covered the cause and treatment of back pain and importantly claimed to be a self help guide.

The author an experienced physiotherapist simply explains the nature of back pain, the psychological aspects of the condition (Tension Related Pain) and more importantly great exercises to perform that help ease pain and also maintain the back.

The instructions were clear with colour pictures showing what needs to be done and "watch points'" for each exercise to highlight good technique. The exercises range from good posture to stretching and to strengthening. It helps to set goals and tasks and I feel an excellent companion for those who suffer from back pain for whom it is often a recurring condition. In this present climate self-management is the way forward and I hope by recommending this book to my patients I can encourage them to self-manage their backs and hopefully reduce relapse. This may in turn reduce my referrals for back and neck pain.

A fantastic book for all back pain sufferers and certainly worthwhile having in your library. "

*Dr Talib Abubacker, GP Luton*